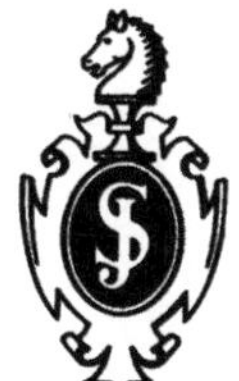

...MCQs... MCQs... MCQs... MCQ

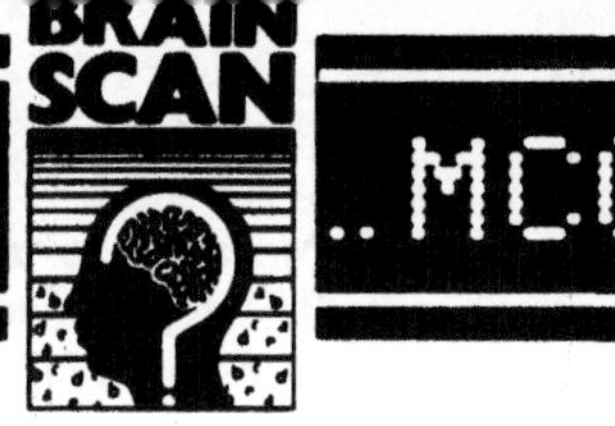

Norman Johnson · Chris Bunker

. . . further MRCP Part I

Springer-Verlag
London Berlin Heidelberg New York
Paris Tokyo Hong Kong
Barcelona Budapest

Norman Johnson, MD, FRCP
The Middlesex Hospital, Mortimer Street,
London W1N 8AA, UK

Christopher Bunker, MD, MRCP
Charing Cross Hospital
London W6 8RF, UK

Publisher's note: the "Brainscan" logo is reproduced by courtesy of The Editor, *Geriatric Medicine*, Modern Medicine GB Ltd.

ISBN-13: 978-3-540-19781-2 e-ISBN-13: 978-1-4471-2005-6
DOI: 10.1007/978-1-4471-2005-6

British Library Cataloguing in Publication Data
A catalogue record for this book is available from the British Library

Typeset by Concept Typesetting Ltd, Salisbury

28/3830-543210 Printed on acid-free paper

Contents

Introduction to MRCP Part I

Multiple choice questions have been a popular way of setting exams for at least 20 years. However fair or unfair they appear to be, they are destined to remain a part of the system. The main reason for their popularity is that they provide a compact method of testing the candidate's knowledge over a very wide field. This is an obvious advantage in a subject such as medicine. Multiple choice questions allow easy and unbiased marking which can be performed rapidly by computer. Computerised marking also facilitates qualitative control of questions and statistical analysis of the exam. In order to discourage wild guessing a heavy penalty is introduced in the form of a negative score for an incorrect answer, which usually results in candidates' answer sheets being returned with a proportion of "don't knows".

The MRCP Part I examination is held three times a year in many centres in the United Kingdom and abroad. A maximum of four attempts at Part I are allowed. Re-entry may be deferred if the candidate fails badly. No set syllabus is published by the Royal Colleges but recently the emphasis of the exam has been on the basic sciences, which will comprise up to 30% of the exam. Sixty multiple choice questions are used from an ever-changing bank of about 4000 questions. A breakdown of the relative distribution of questions is given below.

Topic	*No. of questions asked*
Anatomy	1
Cardiology	4
Clinical pharmacology	5
Dermatology	1
Endocrinology	3
Gastroenterology	3
Genetics	1
Haematology	2 or 3
Immunology or allergy	1
Industrial medicine	1
Infectious diseases	2 or 3
Metabolic disease	2

Musculoskeletal diseases	2
Neurology	4
Ophthalmology	1
Paediatrics	4
Physiology	1
Psychiatry	4
Renal disease	3
Respiratory diseases	4
Reticuloendothelial system	1
Statistics	1
Symptoms and signs	1 or 2
Toxicology	1
Tropical medicine	1 or 0

The exam is essentially competitive, with about the top 30% of candidates passing each time, the passmark therefore being variable. In simple terms, this means that the successful candidate must perform better than the majority of his or her colleagues. Achieving this requires sound knowledge of medicine and basic science, as well as practice in multiple choice question technique.

There is no doubt that at least 12 weeks' serious preparatory work is needed for this exam. A busy clinical job can erode the time spent in the proper preparation which is so necessary for success.

Stage I: This should be a stage of broadly based general reading (see list below), aimed at acquiring good background knowledge.

Stage II: This should be one of using subject-based multiple choice questions to guide detailed reading in areas of weakness. This helps to highlight the fields in which additional reading is valuable. Using multiple choice questions in this way helps the candidate to be guided into those areas on which the College has placed particular emphasis.

Stage III: This stage of preparation for the exam is the most difficult. Many candidates find it hard to take an overall view, but working through multiple choice question papers is probably the best way to polish technique and pick out any final points requiring extra attention. This method also enables one to gain insight into one's own aptitude for multiple choice question exams, which is invaluable when actually sitting the paper. The College quite rightly advises against guessing, but one only learns to assess reasonable certainty by practice and experience.

Bibliography

Brain & Bannister (1992) Clinical neurology, 7th edn. Oxford University Press, Oxford.
Burton JL (1990) Aids to postgraduate medicine, 5th edn. Churchill Livingstone, Edinburgh.
Ellis H (1983) Clinical anatomy, 7th edn. Blackwell Scientific, Oxford.
Forfar JO, Arneil GC (1984) Textbook of paediatrics, vols 1 & 2, 3rd edn. Churchill Livingstone, Edinburgh.
Ganong WF (1989) Review of medical physiology, 14th edn. Lange Medical Publications, Los Altos, California.
Goodman LS, Gilman A (1990) The pharmacological basis of therapeutics, 8th edn. Macmillan, New York.
Harrison's principles of internal medicine (1991) 12th edn. McGraw-Hill, New York.
Johnson NMcI (1990) Respiratory medicine pocket consultant, 2nd edn. Blackwell Scientific, Oxford.
Johnson N, Pozniak A (1986) MRCP Part I. Springer, Berlin, Heidelberg, Hew York.
Johnson N, Bunker C (1988) More MRCP Part I. Springer, Berlin, Heidelberg, New York.
Patten J (1978) Neurological differential diagnosis. Harold Starke, London.
Pocock SJ (1983) Clinical trials: a practical approach. John Wiley & Sons, Chichester
Roitt I et al. (1989) Immunology, 2nd edn. Churchill Livingstone, Edinburgh.
Rubenstein D, Wayne D (1991) Lecture notes on clinical medicine, 4th edn. Blackwell Scientific, Oxford.
Souhami RL, Moxham J (1990) Textbook of medicine. Churchill Livingstone, Edinburgh.
Weatherall DJ (1991) The new genetics and clinical practice, 3rd edn. Oxford University Press, Oxford.
Weatherall DJ, Leadingham JGG, Warrell DA (1987) The Oxford textbook of medicine, 2nd edn. Oxford University Press, Oxford.
Zilva JF, Pannall P (1988) Clinical chemistry in diagnosis and treatment, 5th edn. Lloyd-Luke, London.

Examples of Multiple Choice Questions from the Common Part I MRCP (UK). Royal College of Physicians of Edinburgh, Glasgow and London.
Medicine International 1982 onwards. Abingdon, Oxon OX14 3BR.

Journals: British Medical Journal
British Journal of Hospital Medicine
Hospital Update
The Lancet
New England Journal of Medicine

Addresses of Royal Colleges

Royal College of Physicians of Edinburgh
9 Queen Street
Edinburgh EH2 1JQ

Royal College of Physicians of Glasgow
242 St Vincent Street
Glasgow G2 5RJ

Royal College of Physicians of London
11 St Andrew's Place
Regents Park
London NW1 4LE

How to Use this Book

The passmark given for each paper (with each answer sheet) gives only an arbitrary guide to the performance of previous candidates who have been successful in the membership.

You should use this book as a set of test examinations to be taken in stage III of your revision. By doing so, not only will you gain experience of performing under the stress of a time limit, but you will also be able to assess your strengths and weaknesses. Don't forget to read the questions carefully, check your answers and fill in the answer sheet correctly.

Do these and other questions in your possession over again, coming back repeatedly to those you get wrong.

The Examination

1. You are allowed 2 hours to complete the paper, which is answered on a computer card (see below) with a 2B pencil.

2. Each initial statement or stem has five possible completions, listed (a) to (e).

3. Each of these has to be answered "true", "false" or "don't know" by filling in the appropriate box on the answer sheet.

4. There is no restriction on the number of true or false answers to any question.

Examination 1

All parts of every question must be answered *True* or *False* or *Don't Know* by filling in the box provided. Failure to do so will result in rejection of the answer sheet

EXAMINATION NO.
1

SURNAME

INITIALS

Please use 2B PENCIL only. Rub out all errors thoroughly.
Mark lozenges like ⬬ NOT like this ⊘⊘⊗

T ⬭ = TRUE F ⬭ = FALSE DK ⬭ = DON'T KNOW

	A	B	C	D	E
1	T ⬭ F ⬭ DK ⬭	T ⬭ F ⬭ DK ⬭	T ⬭ F ⬭ DK ⬭	T ⬭ F ⬭ DK ⬭	T ⬭ F ⬭ DK ⬭
2	T ⬭ F ⬭ DK ⬭	T ⬭ F ⬭ DK ⬭	T ⬭ F ⬭ DK ⬭	T ⬭ F ⬭ DK ⬭	T ⬭ F ⬭ DK ⬭
3	T ⬭ F ⬭ DK ⬭	T ⬭ F ⬭ DK ⬭	T ⬭ F ⬭ DK ⬭	T ⬭ F ⬭ DK ⬭	T ⬭ F ⬭ DK ⬭
4	T ⬭ F ⬭ DK ⬭	T ⬭ F ⬭ DK ⬭	T ⬭ F ⬭ DK ⬭	T ⬭ F ⬭ DK ⬭	T ⬭ F ⬭ DK ⬭
5	T ⬭ F ⬭ DK ⬭	T ⬭ F ⬭ DK ⬭	T ⬭ F ⬭ DK ⬭	T ⬭ F ⬭ DK ⬭	T ⬭ F ⬭ DK ⬭
6	T ⬭ F ⬭ DK ⬭	T ⬭ F ⬭ DK ⬭	T ⬭ F ⬭ DK ⬭	T ⬭ F ⬭ DK ⬭	T ⬭ F ⬭ DK ⬭
7	T ⬭ F ⬭ DK ⬭	T ⬭ F ⬭ DK ⬭	T ⬭ F ⬭ DK ⬭	T ⬭ F ⬭ DK ⬭	T ⬭ F ⬭ DK ⬭
8	T ⬭ F ⬭ DK ⬭	T ⬭ F ⬭ DK ⬭	T ⬭ F ⬭ DK ⬭	T ⬭ F ⬭ DK ⬭	T ⬭ F ⬭ DK ⬭
9	T ⬭ F ⬭ DK ⬭	T ⬭ F ⬭ DK ⬭	T ⬭ F ⬭ DK ⬭	T ⬭ F ⬭ DK ⬭	T ⬭ F ⬭ DK ⬭
10	T ⬭ F ⬭ DK ⬭	T ⬭ F ⬭ DK ⬭	T ⬭ F ⬭ DK ⬭	T ⬭ F ⬭ DK ⬭	T ⬭ F ⬭ DK ⬭
11	T ⬭ F ⬭ DK ⬭	T ⬭ F ⬭ DK ⬭	T ⬭ F ⬭ DK ⬭	T ⬭ F ⬭ DK ⬭	T ⬭ F ⬭ DK ⬭
12	T ⬭ F ⬭ DK ⬭	T ⬭ F ⬭ DK ⬭	T ⬭ F ⬭ DK ⬭	T ⬭ F ⬭ DK ⬭	T ⬭ F ⬭ DK ⬭
13	T ⬭ F ⬭ DK ⬭	T ⬭ F ⬭ DK ⬭	T ⬭ F ⬭ DK ⬭	T ⬭ F ⬭ DK ⬭	T ⬭ F ⬭ DK ⬭
14	T ⬭ F ⬭ DK ⬭	T ⬭ F ⬭ DK ⬭	T ⬭ F ⬭ DK ⬭	T ⬭ F ⬭ DK ⬭	T ⬭ F ⬭ DK ⬭
15	T ⬭ F ⬭ DK ⬭	T ⬭ F ⬭ DK ⬭	T ⬭ F ⬭ DK ⬭	T ⬭ F ⬭ DK ⬭	T ⬭ F ⬭ DK ⬭
16	T ⬭ F ⬭ DK ⬭	T ⬭ F ⬭ DK ⬭	T ⬭ F ⬭ DK ⬭	T ⬭ F ⬭ DK ⬭	T ⬭ F ⬭ DK ⬭
17	T ⬭ F ⬭ DK ⬭	T ⬭ F ⬭ DK ⬭	T ⬭ F ⬭ DK ⬭	T ⬭ F ⬭ DK ⬭	T ⬭ F ⬭ DK ⬭
18	T ⬭ F ⬭ DK ⬭	T ⬭ F ⬭ DK ⬭	T ⬭ F ⬭ DK ⬭	T ⬭ F ⬭ DK ⬭	T ⬭ F ⬭ DK ⬭
19	T ⬭ F ⬭ DK ⬭	T ⬭ F ⬭ DK ⬭	T ⬭ F ⬭ DK ⬭	T ⬭ F ⬭ DK ⬭	T ⬭ F ⬭ DK ⬭
20	T ⬭ F ⬭ DK ⬭	T ⬭ F ⬭ DK ⬭	T ⬭ F ⬭ DK ⬭	T ⬭ F ⬭ DK ⬭	T ⬭ F ⬭ DK ⬭
21	T ⬭ F ⬭ DK ⬭	T ⬭ F ⬭ DK ⬭	T ⬭ F ⬭ DK ⬭	T ⬭ F ⬭ DK ⬭	T ⬭ F ⬭ DK ⬭
22	T ⬭ F ⬭ DK ⬭	T ⬭ F ⬭ DK ⬭	T ⬭ F ⬭ DK ⬭	T ⬭ F ⬭ DK ⬭	T ⬭ F ⬭ DK ⬭
23	T ⬭ F ⬭ DK ⬭	T ⬭ F ⬭ DK ⬭	T ⬭ F ⬭ DK ⬭	T ⬭ F ⬭ DK ⬭	T ⬭ F ⬭ DK ⬭
24	T ⬭ F ⬭ DK ⬭	T ⬭ F ⬭ DK ⬭	T ⬭ F ⬭ DK ⬭	T ⬭ F ⬭ DK ⬭	T ⬭ F ⬭ DK ⬭
25	T ⬭ F ⬭ DK ⬭	T ⬭ F ⬭ DK ⬭	T ⬭ F ⬭ DK ⬭	T ⬭ F ⬭ DK ⬭	T ⬭ F ⬭ DK ⬭
26	T ⬭ F ⬭ DK ⬭	T ⬭ F ⬭ DK ⬭	T ⬭ F ⬭ DK ⬭	T ⬭ F ⬭ DK ⬭	T ⬭ F ⬭ DK ⬭
27	T ⬭ F ⬭ DK ⬭	T ⬭ F ⬭ DK ⬭	T ⬭ F ⬭ DK ⬭	T ⬭ F ⬭ DK ⬭	T ⬭ F ⬭ DK ⬭
28	T ⬭ F ⬭ DK ⬭	T ⬭ F ⬭ DK ⬭	T ⬭ F ⬭ DK ⬭	T ⬭ F ⬭ DK ⬭	T ⬭ F ⬭ DK ⬭
29	T ⬭ F ⬭ DK ⬭	T ⬭ F ⬭ DK ⬭	T ⬭ F ⬭ DK ⬭	T ⬭ F ⬭ DK ⬭	T ⬭ F ⬭ DK ⬭
30	T ⬭ F ⬭ DK ⬭	T ⬭ F ⬭ DK ⬭	T ⬭ F ⬭ DK ⬭	T ⬭ F ⬭ DK ⬭	T ⬭ F ⬭ DK ⬭

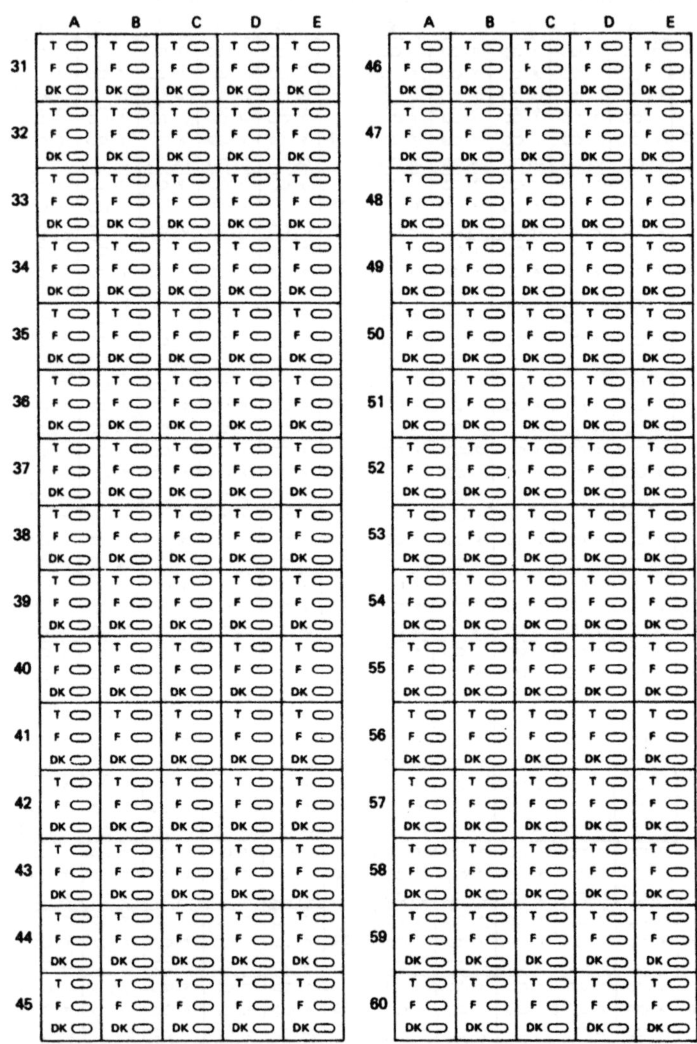

	A	B	C	D	E
31	T F DK	T F DK	T F DK	T F DK	T F DK
32	T F DK	T F DK	T F DK	T F DK	T F DK
33	T F DK	T F DK	T F DK	T F DK	T F DK
34	T F DK	T F DK	T F DK	T F DK	T F DK
35	T F DK	T F DK	T F DK	T F DK	T F DK
36	T F DK	T F DK	T F DK	T F DK	T F DK
37	T F DK	T F DK	T F DK	T F DK	T F DK
38	T F DK	T F DK	T F DK	T F DK	T F DK
39	T F DK	T F DK	T F DK	T F DK	T F DK
40	T F DK	T F DK	T F DK	T F DK	T F DK
41	T F DK	T F DK	T F DK	T F DK	T F DK
42	T F DK	T F DK	T F DK	T F DK	T F DK
43	T F DK	T F DK	T F DK	T F DK	T F DK
44	T F DK	T F DK	T F DK	T F DK	T F DK
45	T F DK	T F DK	T F DK	T F DK	T F DK

	A	B	C	D	E
46	T F DK	T F DK	T F DK	T F DK	T F DK
47	T F DK	T F DK	T F DK	T F DK	T F DK
48	T F DK	T F DK	T F DK	T F DK	T F DK
49	T F DK	T F DK	T F DK	T F DK	T F DK
50	T F DK	T F DK	T F DK	T F DK	T F DK
51	T F DK	T F DK	T F DK	T F DK	T F DK
52	T F DK	T F DK	T F DK	T F DK	T F DK
53	T F DK	T F DK	T F DK	T F DK	T F DK
54	T F DK	T F DK	T F DK	T F DK	T F DK
55	T F DK	T F DK	T F DK	T F DK	T F DK
56	T F DK	T F DK	T F DK	T F DK	T F DK
57	T F DK	T F DK	T F DK	T F DK	T F DK
58	T F DK	T F DK	T F DK	T F DK	T F DK
59	T F DK	T F DK	T F DK	T F DK	T F DK
60	T F DK	T F DK	T F DK	T F DK	T F DK

Q.1.1 HDL hyperlipoproteinaemia is associated with:

a. High total plasma cholesterol levels
b. Athletic training
c. Oestrogen therapy
d. Obesity
e. Increased longevity

Q.1.2 Paradoxical interventricular septal motion may be seen in:

a. Aortic stenosis
b. Myocardial infarction
c. Hypertrophic obstructive cardiomyopathy
d. Right ventricular failure
e. Mitral stenosis

Q.1.3 A diagnosis of myocardial infarction may be excluded if:

a. The ECG is normal
b. There is LBBB (left bundle branch block)
c. The patient is asymptomatic
d. The level of the MB isoenzyme of creatine phosphokinase (MB – CPK) remains normal in the first 24–48 hours
e. The patient has no risk factors for coronary artery disease

Q.1.4 Coronary artery disease is a recognised feature of:

a. Chagas disease
b. Kawasaki disease
c. Elevation of HDL – cholesterol
d. Pseudoxanthoma elasticum
e. Kartagener's syndrome

Q.1.5 Peripheral neuropathy is a recognised feature of:

a. Sarcoidosis
b. Diabetes mellitus
c. Guillain-Barré syndrome
d. Syphilis
e. Amyloidosis

Q.1.6 Pseudomembranous colitis:

a. Is caused by the invasion of the bowel by C. botulism
b. May be caused by clindamycin
c. Responds to metronidazole
d. Never relapses
e. Is associated with characteristic ulceration of the bowel

Q.1.7 Which of the following favour Crohn's disease rather than ulcerative colitis:

a. Rectal involvement
b. Fistulae
c. Loss of colonic haustral pattern
d. Preservation of gland architecture
e. Cobblestoning of mucosa

Q.1.8 The following may cause acute gastritis:

a. Uraemia
b. Prostaglandin E
c. Phenylbutazone
d. Streptococcal septicaemia
e. Histamine

Q.1.9 Proton pump blocking drugs are beneficial in:

a. Asthma
b. Hypertension
c. Bladder neck instability
d. Zollinger–Ellison syndrome
e. Adult respiratory distress syndrome

Q.1.10 Which of the following antibiotics are paired appropriately with a susceptible organism:

a. Erythromycin – *N. meningitidis*
b. Carbenicillin – *S. aureus*
c. Chloramphenicol – *N. gonorrhoea*
d. Gentamicin – *B. fragilis*
e. Mecillinam – *S. aureus*

Q.1.11 Which of the following are recognised causes of megaloblastic anaemia:

a. Tetracyclines
b. Phenytoin
c. Trimethoprim
d. Homocystinuria
e. Thalassaemia major

Q.1.12 Hereditary angioneurotic oedema:

a. Is due to absence of a C_1 inhibitor in the serum
b. Is characterised by multiple, superficial, small swellings of skin
c. Is associated with recurrent abdominal pain
d. May be effectively treated with antihistamines and steroids
e. Is not helped by danazol

Q.1.13 Idiopathic haemochromatosis is characterised by:

a. Autosomal dominant inheritance
b. High serum iron and low ferritin
c. Increased urine iron excretion after desferrioxamine
d. Hyperuricaemia
e. Frequent onset in adolescence

Q.1.14 Basophilic stippling of red cells is a recognised feature of:

a. Thalassaemia
b. Myelofibrosis
c. Lead poisoning
d. Post splenectomy
e. Renal failure

Q.1.15 Which of the following are recognised radiological signs of sickle cell disease:

a. Splenic calcification
b. Bone cysts
c. Coarse trabecular pattern of long bones
d. Osteoporosis
e. Soft tissue calcification of the fingertips

Q.1.16 Which of the following are causes of a non-thrombocytopenic purpura:

a. Vitamin B12 deficiency
b. Haemangioma
c. Scurvy
d. Paraproteinaemia
e. Amyloidosis

Q.1.17 Recognised causes of bronchial carcinoma include:

a. Cadmium exposure
b. Pleural plaques
c. Nickel exposure
d. Chronic heroin abuse
e. Retrovirus infection

Q.1.18 In the chemotherapy of pulmonary tuberculosis:

a. Rifampicin is bacteriostatic
b. Ethambutol is bacteriocidal
c. Pyridoxine is teratogenic
d. Pyrazinamide penetrates poorly into CSF
e. The recommended treatment in pregnancy is identical to that in non-pregnant patients

Q.1.19 Pulmonary granuloma are characteristic of:

a. Histoplasmosis
b. Berylliosis
c. Histiocytosis
d. Churg-Strauss syndrome
e. Goodpasture's syndrome

Q.1.20 Which of the following are characteristic features of bronchial carcinoid tumours:

a. Superior vena cava obstruction
b. Radiological evidence of calcification
c. Recurrent chest infections
d. Haemoptysis with normal chest x-ray
e. Weight loss

Q.1.21 In HIV infected individuals which of the following are common:

a. Shingles
b. Primary intrathoracic lymphoma
c. *Helicobacter pylorii* infection
d. Bacterial pneumonias
e. Listeriosis

Q.1.22 Deficiencies of which of the following vitamins are correctly paired with their clinical consequences:

a. Thiamine – Beri beri
b. Niacin – Pellagra
c. Riboflavin – Bitot's spots
d. Thiamine – Ophthalmoplegia
e. Pyridoxine – Night blindness

Q.1.23 Characteristic features of acute tubular necrosis include:

a. Enlarged, oedematous kidneys
b. Macroscopic haematuria
c. Prolonged oliguria
d. Hypertension
e. Asterixis

Q.1.24 In renal osteodystrophy:

a. Renal 1α hydroxylase is inhibited by hyperphosphataemia
b. Parathyroidectomy is indicated for intractable pruritis
c. 1,25 hydroxy vitamin D levels are low
d. Plasma calcium may be normal
e. There is improvement with dialysis

Q.1.25 C reactive protein estimation may be more helpful than an ESR in which of these diseases:

a. SLE
b. Graft versus host disease
c. Lymphoma
d. Leukaemia
e. Pyelonephritis

Q.1.26 Clinical associations of the lupus anticoagulant include:

a. Tissue eosinophilia
b. False positive syphilis serology
c. Recurrent abortion
d. Peripheral neuropathy
e. Raynaud's phenomenon

Q.1.27 Bony metastases:

a. Commonly occur in prostate cancer
b. Most commonly cause hypercalcaemia in thyroid and kidney cancer
c. Are commonly osteosclerotic in lung cancer
d. Respond poorly to local radiotherapy
e. With osteolytic activity may be suppressed by aspirin

Q.1.28 The differential diagnosis of a lymphocytic CSF includes:

a. Lyme disease
b. Sarcoidosis
c. Tuberculosis
d. Cryptococcal meningitis
e. Syphilis

Q.1.29 Which of the following are acute phase reactants:

a. Alpha I antitrypsin
b. C reactive protein
c. Type VII collagen
d. Ferritin
e. Renin

Q.1.30 Raised serum alkaline phosphatase concentration is characteristically associated with:

a. Hypophosphatasia
b. Osteomalacia
c. Myeloma
d. Benign prostatic hypertrophy
e. Paget's disease

Q.1.31 Which of the following thyroid function tests are useful in the condition with which they are paired:

a. TSH – Neonatal screening for cretinism
b. TRH – Thyroid eye disease
c. T3 – Hypothyroidism
d. Thyroid ultrasound – Goitre
e. T4 – Thyrotoxicosis

Q.1.32 Which of the following are recognised causes of stones in the urinary tract:

a. Dehydration
b. Medullary sponge kidneys
c. Polycystic kidneys
d. Hyperuricaemia
e. Renal tubular acidosis

Q.1.33 Which of the following are recognised signs of cervical spondylosis:

a. Nystagmus
b. Rombergism
c. Upgoing plantars
d. Absent knee jerks
e. Grasp reflex

Q.1.34 In tuberous sclerosis:

a. Most newly identified patients represent new mutations
b. 80% of patients have fits
c. Visceral lesions (other than cerebral) often cause symptoms
d. Mental handicap is an invariable association
e. The adenoma sebaceum may respond to argon-laser treatment

Q.1.35 Which of the following are characteristic of temporal lobe lesions:

a. Ataxia
b. Incontinence
c. Grasp reflex
d. Memory impairment
e. Hyperphagia

Q.1.36 The incidence of childhood cerebral palsy can be reduced by:

a. Rubella immunisation of adolescent girls
b. Prevention of rhesus iso-immunisation
c. Caesarean section replacing hazardous forceps deliveries
d. Genetic counselling
e. Antenatal screening for neural tube defects

Q.1.37 Recognised pulmonary complications of rheumatoid arthritis include:

a. Lymphangioleiomyomatosis
b. Stridor
c. Fibrosing alveolitis
d. Emphysema
e. Decreased functional residual capacity (of the lung)

Q.1.38 Pencillamine nephropathy in rheumatoid arthritis:

a. Rarely occurs in the first year of treatment
b. May be avoided by lower doses
c. Is usually associated with resolution of proteinuria after stopping treatment
d. May result in the nephrotic syndrome
e. Is usually associated with membranous glomerulonephritis on renal biopsy

Q.1.39 The American Rheumatism Assocation criteria for the diagnosis of systemic lupus erythematosus include:

a. Discoid rash
b. Photosensitivity
c. Erosive arthritis
d. Hepatosplenomegaly
e. Oral ulceration

Q.1.40 In Reiter's syndrome:

a. Over half of patients are symptom free after six months
b. Early antibiotic treatment diminishes the severity of the arthritis
c. Local steroid injections may alleviate enthesopathy
d. HLA B27 positivity points to a poorer prognosis
e. Gold salts have been shown to be effective in severe cases

Q.1.41 The differential diagnosis of sacro-iliitis includes:

a. Psoriasis
b. Brucellosis
c. Ochronosis
d. Familial Mediterranean fever
e. SLE

Q.1.42 In hepatitis B infection:

a. The e antigen is the first to appear in the serum
b. RNA directed DNA synthesis plays an essential role in the life cycle of the virus
c. The carrier state is established in approximately 10%
d. Post-exposure passive immunisation is best administered in the first seven days
e. The virus is spread exclusively by blood or blood products

Q.1.43 In leprosy:

a. There may be transplacental transmission
b. The lepromin test is positive in the lepromatous type
c. Depigmented patches are typically hyperaesthetic
d. The commonest cause of death in the lepromatous type is renal failure
e. Thalidomide is useful

Q.1.44 Endogenous pyrogens include:

a. Interleukin 1
b. Tumour necrosis factor
c. Interferon γ
d. Prostaglandin E2
e. Insulin

Q.1.45 Ciprofloxacin:

a. Is useful for chlamydial infections
b. Is used to eradicate the carrier state in typhoid
c. May cause urticarial rashes
d. Is a fluoroquinolone
e. Is cheaper than trimethoprim

Q.1.46 Drugs used in the treatment of epilepsy:

a. Phenobarbitone is a first line drug for grand mal seizures
b. Sodium valproate is effective in myoclonic epilepsy
c. Vigabratin produces a psychosis in up to 50% of patients treated
d. Carbamazepine can cause blood dyscrasias
e. Phenytoin toxicity is associated with an irreversible cerebellar syndrome

Q.1.47 Which of the following drugs are recognised causes of psychosis:

a. Steroids
b. Retinoids
c. Amitriptyline
d. Metronidazole
e. Phenothiazines

Q.1.48 Which of the following are used to stage malignant diseases:

a. Jellinek classification
b. Karnowsky performance scale
c. TNM classification
d. Ann Arbor system
e. Rye classification

Q.1.49 Recognised causes of hypercalcaemia include:

a. Thiazide therapy
b. Addison's disease
c. Thyrotoxicosis
d. Long term immobility
e. Pseudohypoparathyroidism

Q.1.50 Recognised causes of hyperprolactinaemia include:

a. Ovarian carcinoma
b. Congenital adrenal hyperplasia
c. Bromocriptine
d. Thyrotoxicosis
e. Chlorpromazine

Q.1.51 Elevation of the glycosylated Hb level is associated with:

a. Renal failure
b. Alcohol abuse
c. Pregnancy
d. Ketoacidosis
e. Iron deficiency

Q.1.52 Which of the following are recognised treatments for Cushing's disease:

a. Transphenoidal yttrium 90 insertion
b. Bilateral adrenalectomy
c. Transphenoidal adenectomy
d. External beam pituitary irradiation
e. Transphenoidal hypophysectomy

Q.1.53 Hypoglycaemia may result from:

a. Cerebellar haemangioma
b. Glucagonoma
c. Uterine fibroids
d. Mesothelioma
e. Choriocarcinoma

Q.1.54 Which of the following immunoglobulins and their properties are correctly paired:

a. IgA – binds to mast cells
b. IgD – five basic subunits
c. IgE – 10% of total immunoglobulins
d. IgG – four subclasses
e. IgM – crosses placenta

Q.1.55 An elevated T helper:suppressor cell ratio is characteristic of:

a. Renal transplant rejection
b. AIDS
c. Acute graft versus host disease
d. Chronic graft versus host disease
e. SLE

Q.1.56 Which of the following drugs characteristically give rise to physical dependence:

a. Phenobarbitone
b. Amphetamine
c. Alcohol
d. Morphine
e. Diazepam

Q.1.57 Sex linked inheritance:

a. Never causes disease in female carriers
b. Is excluded by direct male to male transmission
c. Is responsible for most of the commonest single gene disorders
d. Carrier status detection is important for all sisters of affected boys
e. Is responsible for Anderson-Fabry disease

Q.1.58 Which of the following are causes of an acute toxic confusional state:

a. Benign intracranial hypertension
b. Syringobulbia
c. Temporal arteritis
d. Hypercapnia
e. Systemic lupus erythematosus

Q.1.59 Which of the following muscles and root values are correctly paired:

a. C5 – finger flexors
b. C6 – deltoid
c. C7 – biceps
d. L4 – peronei
e. L5 – thigh adductors

Q.1.60 Flapping tremor of the hands is a recognised feature of:

a. Salbutamol therapy
b. Steroid psychosis
c. Liver failure
d. Parkinson's disease
e. Cerebellar degeneration

Examination 2

All parts of every question must be answered *True* or *False* or *Don't Know* by filling in the box provided. Failure to do so will result in rejection of the answer sheet

EXAMINATION NO.
2

SURNAME

[ ]

INITIALS

[ ]

Please use 2B PENCIL only. Rub out all errors thoroughly.
Mark lozenges like ⬬ NOT like this ⊄ ⊄ ⊄

T ⬭ = TRUE F ⬭ = FALSE DK ⬭ = DON'T KNOW

	A	B	C	D	E
1	T F DK	T F DK	T F DK	T F DK	T F DK
2	T F DK	T F DK	T F DK	T F DK	T F DK
3	T F DK	T F DK	T F DK	T F DK	T F DK
4	T F DK	T F DK	T F DK	T F DK	T F DK
5	T F DK	T F DK	T F DK	T F DK	T F DK
6	T F DK	T F DK	T F DK	T F DK	T F DK
7	T F DK	T F DK	T F DK	T F DK	T F DK
8	T F DK	T F DK	T F DK	T F DK	T F DK
9	T F DK	T F DK	T F DK	T F DK	T F DK
10	T F DK	T F DK	T F DK	T F DK	T F DK
11	T F DK	T F DK	T F DK	T F DK	T F DK
12	T F DK	T F DK	T F DK	T F DK	T F DK
13	T F DK	T F DK	T F DK	T F DK	T F DK
14	T F DK	T F DK	T F DK	T F DK	T F DK
15	T F DK	T F DK	T F DK	T F DK	T F DK

	A	B	C	D	E
16	T F DK	T F DK	T F DK	T F DK	T F DK
17	T F DK	T F DK	T F DK	T F DK	T F DK
18	T F DK	T F DK	T F DK	T F DK	T F DK
19	T F DK	T F DK	T F DK	T F DK	T F DK
20	T F DK	T F DK	T F DK	T F DK	T F DK
21	T F DK	T F DK	T F DK	T F DK	T F DK
22	T F DK	T F DK	T F DK	T F DK	T F DK
23	T F DK	T F DK	T F DK	T F DK	T F DK
24	T F DK	T F DK	T F DK	T F DK	T F DK
25	T F DK	T F DK	T F DK	T F DK	T F DK
26	T F DK	T F DK	T F DK	T F DK	T F DK
27	T F DK	T F DK	T F DK	T F DK	T F DK
28	T F DK	T F DK	T F DK	T F DK	T F DK
29	T F DK	T F DK	T F DK	T F DK	T F DK
30	T F DK	T F DK	T F DK	T F DK	T F DK

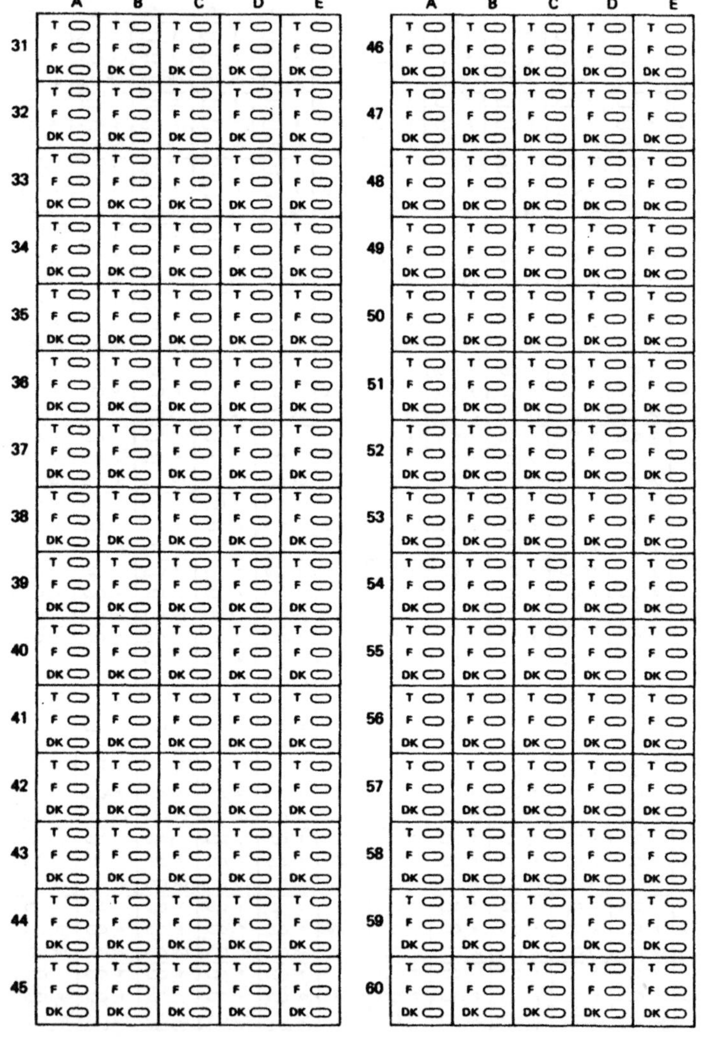

	A	B	C	D	E
31	T F DK	T F DK	T F DK	T F DK	T F DK
32	T F DK	T F DK	T F DK	T F DK	T F DK
33	T F DK	T F DK	T F DK	T F DK	T F DK
34	T F DK	T F DK	T F DK	T F DK	T F DK
35	T F DK	T F DK	T F DK	T F DK	T F DK
36	T F DK	T F DK	T F DK	T F DK	T F DK
37	T F DK	T F DK	T F DK	T F DK	T F DK
38	T F DK	T F DK	T F DK	T F DK	T F DK
39	T F DK	T F DK	T F DK	T F DK	T F DK
40	T F DK	T F DK	T F DK	T F DK	T F DK
41	T F DK	T F DK	T F DK	T F DK	T F DK
42	T F DK	T F DK	T F DK	T F DK	T F DK
43	T F DK	T F DK	T F DK	T F DK	T F DK
44	T F DK	T F DK	T F DK	T F DK	T F DK
45	T F DK	T F DK	T F DK	T F DK	T F DK

	A	B	C	D	E
46	T F DK	T F DK	T F DK	T F DK	T F DK
47	T F DK	T F DK	T F DK	T F DK	T F DK
48	T F DK	T F DK	T F DK	T F DK	T F DK
49	T F DK	T F DK	T F DK	T F DK	T F DK
50	T F DK	T F DK	T F DK	T F DK	T F DK
51	T F DK	T F DK	T F DK	T F DK	T F DK
52	T F DK	T F DK	T F DK	T F DK	T F DK
53	T F DK	T F DK	T F DK	T F DK	T F DK
54	T F DK	T F DK	T F DK	T F DK	T F DK
55	T F DK	T F DK	T F DK	T F DK	T F DK
56	T F DK	T F DK	T F DK	T F DK	T F DK
57	T F DK	T F DK	T F DK	T F DK	T F DK
58	T F DK	T F DK	T F DK	T F DK	T F DK
59	T F DK	T F DK	T F DK	T F DK	T F DK
60	T F DK	T F DK	T F DK	T F DK	T F DK

Q.2.1 Myocardial infarction may be caused by:

a. Myxoedema
b. Aortic valve stenosis
c. Mitral stenosis
d. HIV infection
e. Coronary angioplasty

Q.2.2 Cardiomyopathy is a recognised feature of:

a. Tuberculosis
b. Pancreatitis
c. Chagas disease
d. Sarcoidosis
e. Pregnancy

Q.2.3 A false positive exercise ECG may be found in:

a. Females
b. Left bundle branch block
c. Digoxin therapy
d. Hypokalaemia
e. Anaemia

Q.2.4 Complications of Swan–Ganz catheterisation are recognised to:

a. Include pulmonary infarction
b. Include asthma
c. Be usually fatal
d. Be commoner in the first 24-hours
e. Include sepsis

Q.2.5 Chylous ascites may be caused by:

a. Budd–Chiari syndrome
b. Tuberculosis
c. Hepatoma
d. Nephrotic syndrome
e. Hodgkin's lymphoma

Q.2.6 Which of the following are histological features of alcoholic liver disease:

a. Piecemeal necrosis
b. Kupffer cell hyperplasia
c. Mononuclear infiltrate of portal tract
d. Pericellular fibrosis
e. Giant mitochondria

Q.2.7 Which of the following are recognised causes of vomiting:

a. Digoxin therapy
b. Erythromelalgia
c. Hypercalcaemia
d. Morphine therapy
e. Migraine

Q.2.8 Which of the following are recognised causes of pancreatitis:

a. Hypocalcaemia
b. Acute renal failure
c. Portal vein thrombosis
d. Hypoglycaemia
e. Paralytic ileus

Q.2.9 Which of these are recognised associations:

a. Methotrexate and baldness
b. Azathioprine and cholestasis
c. Gold and leucopenia
d. Cyclophosphamide and haematuria
e. Cyclosporin and lymphoma

Q.2.10 Erythromycin is a recognised cause of:

a. Pericarditis
b. Goitre
c. Eosinophilia
d. Jaundice
e. Gout

Q.2.11 Zidovudine (AZT) is recognised to cause:

a. Abdominal pain
b. Insomnia
c. Hyperuricaemia
d. Angina
e. Leucopaenia

Q.2.12 Cardiac afterload is reduced by:

a. Phentolamine
b. Nifedipine
c. Prazosin
d. Morphine
e. Minoxidil

Q.2.13 Which of the following favours a diagnosis of secondary polycythaemia:

a. Normal platelet count
b. PCV greater than 55%
c. Splenomegaly
d. Oxygen saturation > 96%
e. Elevated P_a CO_2

Q.2.14 The following are recognised causes of iron deficiency anaemia:

a. Cirrhosis
b. Crohn's disease
c. Tropical sprue
d. Polycythaemia rubra vera
e. *Necator americanus* infection

Q.2.15 Acute renal failure following a Lancefield Group A streptococcal infection is characteristically associated with:

a. Hypotension
b. Haematuria
c. Hyperkalaemia
d. Renal colic
e. Erythema nodosum

Q.2.16 Chronic renal failure:

a. Causes a metabolic alkalosis
b. Predisposes to renal carcinoma
c. Promotes subperiosteal bone erosion
d. Reduces the urine volume
e. Causes skin cancer

Q.2.17 Recognised precipitants of acute asthma include:

a. Cold air
b. Sex
c. Analgesics
d. Desensitisation
e. Leukotriene antagonists

Q.2.18 Supplemental (domiciliary) oxygen therapy:

a. Must be given at 2 litres/min for 15 hours a day to reduce mortality in hypoxic chronic airflow obstruction
b. Is most cheaply delivered by oxygen concentrator
c. Is contraindicated by continued smoking
d. Is prescribable on Form FP10
e. Is not indicated in conditions other than hypoxaemic chronic airflow obstruction

Q.2.19 Recognised causes of pulmonary eosinophilia include:

a. Loeffler's syndrome
b. Polyarteritis nodosa
c. *Aspergillus fumigatus*
d. Nitrofurantoin therapy
e. Churg Strauss syndrome

Q.2.20 Drugs which are recognised to cause asthma include:

a. Aspirin
b. Propranolol
c. Azathioprine
d. Cyclophosphamide
e. Diamorphine

Q.2.21 Which of the following are accepted drug combinations:

a. Cyclosporin and azathioprine
b. Dithranol and topical steroid
c. Digoxin and potassium supplements
d. Chlorpropamide and glibenclamide
e. Ampicillin and flucloxacillin

Q.2.22 LSD is:

a. 4000 times more potent than mescaline
b. Effective three hours after ingestion
c. Associated with synaesthesias
d. Only efficacious in tablet form
e. Causes parasympathetic stimulation

Q.2.23 Purpura is a characteristic feature of septicaemia due to:

a. Leptospirae
b. Propionobacteriae
c. Pneumococci
d. Meningococci
e. Staphylococci

Q.2.24 Recognised features of chronic heavy ethanol consumption include:

a. Polydipsia
b. Nystagmus
c. Painless rib fractures
d. Heberden's nodes
e. Cardiomyopathy

Q.2.25 The following diseases have been mapped to the chromosomes with which they are paired:

a. Huntingdon's chorea – 4p
b. Cystic fibrosis – 7q
c. Polycystic kidneys – 16p
d. Neurofibromatosis – 17
e. Polyposis coli – 5q

Q.2.26 A grossly elevated ESR (>100mm/h) may be a feature of:

a. Uraemia
b. Hypofibrinogenaemia
c. Profound anaemia
d. Hypogammaglobulinaemia
e. Polyarteritis nodosa

Q.2.27 Which of the following findings would support the diagnosis of systemic lupus erythematosus:

a. Photophobia
b. Thrombocytopaenia
c. Pericardial pain
d. Heavy proteinuria
e. Low vital capacity

Q.2.28 Recognised features of gluten-sensitive enteropathy include:

a. Delayed puberty
b. Bone pain
c. Jejunal villous atrophy
d. Anorexia
e. Milk intolerance

Q.2.29 Hypomagnesaemia is a recognised cause of:

a. Refractory arrhythmias
b. Muscle weakness
c. Digoxin toxicity
d. Persistent diarrhoea
e. Myalgic encephalomyelitis

Q.2.30 Diabetic nephropathy:

a. Causes end stage renal failure in 10 per million in the UK per year
b. Occurs in 40% of patients with diabetes
c. Is associated with cigarette smoking
d. Is not associated with cardiovascular morbidity and mortality
e. Is commoner in caucasians

Q.2.31 Depressive illness occurring in a man of 65:

a. Responds poorly to tricyclics
b. Can resemble dementia
c. Is usually due to organic diseases
d. Rarely leads to suicide
e. May respond to electro-convulsive therapy (ECT)

Q.2.32 Solvent abuse is a recognised cause of:

a. Over 100 deaths a year in the UK
b. Perioral eczema
c. Delusions
d. Cardiac dysrhythmias
e. Dependence

Q.2.33 Causes of loss of abdominal reflexes include:

a. Multiple sclerosis
b. Friedrich's ataxia
c. Obesity
d. Spinal cord lesions
e. Poliomyelitis

Q.2.34 Which of the following statements concerning intracranial tumours are true:

a. Medulloblastoma rarely metastasise
b. Meningioma is radiosensitive
c. Craniopharyngioma is more prevalent in children than in adults
d. Death is usually due to intraventricular haemorrhage
e. Acoustic Schwannoma is associated with neurofibromatosis

Q.2.35 Alzheimer's disease is:

a. The most common form of dementia in the UK
b. Due to raw beef ingestion
c. Associated with neurofibrillary tangles
d. Due to dopaminergic neuronal loss
e. Common in Down's syndrome

Q.2.36 Which of the following are recognised causes of a scarring conjunctivitis:

a. Sjögren's syndrome
b. Erythema multiforme
c. Rosacea
d. Ionising radiation
e. Trachoma

Q.2.37 Behçet's disease is often associated with which of the following:

a. Painless ulceration
b. Ocular problems
c. Haemoptysis
d. Long term joint disability
e. HLA B27

Q.2.38 Oral gold treatment in rheumatoid arthritis:

a. Obviates the need for regular blood tests
b. Is much less effective than injectable gold
c. Improves the long-term outcome of the disease
d. Produces side effects more commonly than injectable gold
e. Is cheaper than injectable gold

Q.2.39 Colchicine:

a. Causes constipation
b. Causes red discolouration of the tongue
c. Is used in familial Mediterranean fever
d. Affects cellular microtubular function
e. Is a treatment for *Herpes zoster*

Q.2.40 Characteristic features of childhood autism include:

a. Above average intelligence
b. Neurofibromata
c. A predisposition to epilepsy
d. Port wine stain
e. Absence of affectionate relationships

Q.2.41 Most children aged 15 months:

a. Can read three words
b. Are continent of urine at night
c. Walk with one hand being held
d. Say two or three words
e. Transfer objects from one hand to another

Q.2.42 Which of the following infectious diseases are recognised to present with dysphagia:

a. Tetanus
b. Diphtheria
c. Poliomyelitis
d. Botulism
e. Syphilis

Q.2.43 Fever and focal neurological signs are characteristic of:

a. Listeriosis
b. Falciparum malaria
c. Herpes simplex encephalitis
d. Typhoid
e. Lyme disease

Q.2.44 Arthropathy and a rash in children are characteristic features of:

a. Parvovirus B19 infection
b. Rubella
c. Still's disease
d. Schistosomiasis
e. Anorexia nervosa

Q.2.45 In travellers' diarrhoea:

a. Routine microbiological analysis is usually negative
b. About 5% of cases are due to cryptosporidial infection
c. Giardiasis causes holidays to be spoilt
d. Bloody stools mean that *Entamoeba coli* should be excluded
e. Diphenyloxalate and atropine is rational treatment for shigellosis

Q.2.46 Neurological disturbance is recognised to occur in:

a. Trichinosis
b. Trichuriasis
c. Toxoplasmosis
d. Toxocariasis
e. Taeniasis

Q.2.47 Which of the following antimicrobials are useful in the management of gram negative sepsis:

a. Penicillin G
b. Amikacin
c. Vancomycin
d. Teicoplanin
e. Aztreonam

Q.2.48 Gram negative bacteria in the CSF are characteristic of infection with:

a. *Escherichia coli*
b. *Listeria monocytogenes*
c. *Haemophilus influenzae*
d. *Neisseria meningitidis*
e. *Propionibacterium acnes*

Q.2.49 Ziehl–Nielsen staining can be used to assist in the diagnosis of:

a. *Mycobacteria leprae*
b. Cryptosporidium
c. *Nocardia asteroides*
d. *Staphylococcus aureus*
e. *Candida albicans*

Q.2.50 Tardive dyskinesia:

a. Occurs in 50% of patients on long-term neuroleptic therapy
b. Is cured in all patients by the withdrawal of the causative agent
c. May be caused by metaclopramide
d. Does not occur in children
e. Is readily treated with anticholinergic drugs

Q.2.51 Elevated plasma renin activity is found in:

a. Bartter's syndrome
b. Addison's disease
c. Old age
d. Malignant hypertension
e. Conn's syndrome

Q.2.52 Clinical features of a prolactinoma include:

a. Dysfunctional uterine bleeding
b. Infertility
c. Increased libido
d. Visual field defect
e. Diabetes mellitus

Q.2.53 Apparent insulin resistance in a diabetic may result from:

a. Addison's disease
b. Hyperkalaemia
c. Elevated C peptide levels
d. Anorexia
e. Insulin

Q.2.54 Which of the following tend to increase the glycosylated haemoglobin:

a. Third trimester of pregnancy
b. Iron deficiency
c. Aspirin ingestion
d. Renal failure
e. Haemolysis

Q.2.55 Transitional cell carcinoma of the bladder:

a. May be related to phenacetin ingestion
b. Is particularly suggested by clots in the urine
c. Is commoner in women
d. Is related to smoking
e. Is curable by chemotherapy

Q.2.56 Which of the following diseases are associated with HLA, B8, DR3:

a. Myasthenia gravis
b. Ankylosing spondylitis
c. Psoriatic arthritis
d. Behçet's syndrome
e. Chronic active hepatitis (HBSAg negative)

Q.2.57 The following are recognised causes of iritis:

a. Diabetes mellitus
b. Brucellosis
c. Behçet's disease
d. Toxocariasis
e. Gonorrhoea

Q.2.58 Depression is a recognised complication of:

a. Variegate porphyria
b. Clonidine
c. Hepatitis
d. Terfenadine
e. The menopause

Q.2.59 Cigarette smoking is associated with:

a. Decreased heart rate
b. Increased threshold to ventricular fibrillation
c. Increased platelet adhesion
d. Decreased HDL-cholesterol
e. Decreased haematocrit

Q.2.60 In which of the following conditions do tendon nodules occur:

a. Tophaceous gout
b. Hypercholesterolaemia
c. Myxoedema
d. Ochronosis
e. Porphyria

Examination 3

All parts of every question must be answered *True* or *False* or *Don't Know* by filling in the box provided. Failure to do so will result in rejection of the answer sheet

EXAMINATION NO.
3

SURNAME

INITIALS

Please use 2B PENCIL only. Rub out all errors thoroughly.
Mark lozenges like ⬬ NOT like this ⊄⊄⊄

T ⬭ = TRUE F ⬭ = FALSE DK ⬭ = DON'T KNOW

	A	B	C	D	E
1	T ⬭ F ⬭ DK ⬭	T ⬭ F ⬭ DK ⬭	T ⬭ F ⬭ DK ⬭	T ⬭ F ⬭ DK ⬭	T ⬭ F ⬭ DK ⬭
2	T ⬭ F ⬭ DK ⬭	T ⬭ F ⬭ DK ⬭	T ⬭ F ⬭ DK ⬭	T ⬭ F ⬭ DK ⬭	T ⬭ F ⬭ DK ⬭
3	T ⬭ F ⬭ DK ⬭	T ⬭ F ⬭ DK ⬭	T ⬭ F ⬭ DK ⬭	T ⬭ F ⬭ DK ⬭	T ⬭ F ⬭ DK ⬭
4	T ⬭ F ⬭ DK ⬭	T ⬭ F ⬭ DK ⬭	T ⬭ F ⬭ DK ⬭	T ⬭ F ⬭ DK ⬭	T ⬭ F ⬭ DK ⬭
5	T ⬭ F ⬭ DK ⬭	T ⬭ F ⬭ DK ⬭	T ⬭ F ⬭ DK ⬭	T ⬭ F ⬭ DK ⬭	T ⬭ F ⬭ DK ⬭
6	T ⬭ F ⬭ DK ⬭	T ⬭ F ⬭ DK ⬭	T ⬭ F ⬭ DK ⬭	T ⬭ F ⬭ DK ⬭	T ⬭ F ⬭ DK ⬭
7	T ⬭ F ⬭ DK ⬭	T ⬭ F ⬭ DK ⬭	T ⬭ F ⬭ DK ⬭	T ⬭ F ⬭ DK ⬭	T ⬭ F ⬭ DK ⬭
8	T ⬭ F ⬭ DK ⬭	T ⬭ F ⬭ DK ⬭	T ⬭ F ⬭ DK ⬭	T ⬭ F ⬭ DK ⬭	T ⬭ F ⬭ DK ⬭
9	T ⬭ F ⬭ DK ⬭	T ⬭ F ⬭ DK ⬭	T ⬭ F ⬭ DK ⬭	T ⬭ F ⬭ DK ⬭	T ⬭ F ⬭ DK ⬭
10	T ⬭ F ⬭ DK ⬭	T ⬭ F ⬭ DK ⬭	T ⬭ F ⬭ DK ⬭	T ⬭ F ⬭ DK ⬭	T ⬭ F ⬭ DK ⬭
11	T ⬭ F ⬭ DK ⬭	T ⬭ F ⬭ DK ⬭	T ⬭ F ⬭ DK ⬭	T ⬭ F ⬭ DK ⬭	T ⬭ F ⬭ DK ⬭
12	T ⬭ F ⬭ DK ⬭	T ⬭ F ⬭ DK ⬭	T ⬭ F ⬭ DK ⬭	T ⬭ F ⬭ DK ⬭	T ⬭ F ⬭ DK ⬭
13	T ⬭ F ⬭ DK ⬭	T ⬭ F ⬭ DK ⬭	T ⬭ F ⬭ DK ⬭	T ⬭ F ⬭ DK ⬭	T ⬭ F ⬭ DK ⬭
14	T ⬭ F ⬭ DK ⬭	T ⬭ F ⬭ DK ⬭	T ⬭ F ⬭ DK ⬭	T ⬭ F ⬭ DK ⬭	T ⬭ F ⬭ DK ⬭
15	T ⬭ F ⬭ DK ⬭	T ⬭ F ⬭ DK ⬭	T ⬭ F ⬭ DK ⬭	T ⬭ F ⬭ DK ⬭	T ⬭ F ⬭ DK ⬭

	A	B	C	D	E
16	T ⬭ F ⬭ DK ⬭	T ⬭ F ⬭ DK ⬭	T ⬭ F ⬭ DK ⬭	T ⬭ F ⬭ DK ⬭	T ⬭ F ⬭ DK ⬭
17	T ⬭ F ⬭ DK ⬭	T ⬭ F ⬭ DK ⬭	T ⬭ F ⬭ DK ⬭	T ⬭ F ⬭ DK ⬭	T ⬭ F ⬭ DK ⬭
18	T ⬭ F ⬭ DK ⬭	T ⬭ F ⬭ DK ⬭	T ⬭ F ⬭ DK ⬭	T ⬭ F ⬭ DK ⬭	T ⬭ F ⬭ DK ⬭
19	T ⬭ F ⬭ DK ⬭	T ⬭ F ⬭ DK ⬭	T ⬭ F ⬭ DK ⬭	T ⬭ F ⬭ DK ⬭	T ⬭ F ⬭ DK ⬭
20	T ⬭ F ⬭ DK ⬭	T ⬭ F ⬭ DK ⬭	T ⬭ F ⬭ DK ⬭	T ⬭ F ⬭ DK ⬭	T ⬭ F ⬭ DK ⬭
21	T ⬭ F ⬭ DK ⬭	T ⬭ F ⬭ DK ⬭	T ⬭ F ⬭ DK ⬭	T ⬭ F ⬭ DK ⬭	T ⬭ F ⬭ DK ⬭
22	T ⬭ F ⬭ DK ⬭	T ⬭ F ⬭ DK ⬭	T ⬭ F ⬭ DK ⬭	T ⬭ F ⬭ DK ⬭	T ⬭ F ⬭ DK ⬭
23	T ⬭ F ⬭ DK ⬭	T ⬭ F ⬭ DK ⬭	T ⬭ F ⬭ DK ⬭	T ⬭ F ⬭ DK ⬭	T ⬭ F ⬭ DK ⬭
24	T ⬭ F ⬭ DK ⬭	T ⬭ F ⬭ DK ⬭	T ⬭ F ⬭ DK ⬭	T ⬭ F ⬭ DK ⬭	T ⬭ F ⬭ DK ⬭
25	T ⬭ F ⬭ DK ⬭	T ⬭ F ⬭ DK ⬭	T ⬭ F ⬭ DK ⬭	T ⬭ F ⬭ DK ⬭	T ⬭ F ⬭ DK ⬭
26	T ⬭ F ⬭ DK ⬭	T ⬭ F ⬭ DK ⬭	T ⬭ F ⬭ DK ⬭	T ⬭ F ⬭ DK ⬭	T ⬭ F ⬭ DK ⬭
27	T ⬭ F ⬭ DK ⬭	T ⬭ F ⬭ DK ⬭	T ⬭ F ⬭ DK ⬭	T ⬭ F ⬭ DK ⬭	T ⬭ F ⬭ DK ⬭
28	T ⬭ F ⬭ DK ⬭	T ⬭ F ⬭ DK ⬭	T ⬭ F ⬭ DK ⬭	T ⬭ F ⬭ DK ⬭	T ⬭ F ⬭ DK ⬭
29	T ⬭ F ⬭ DK ⬭	T ⬭ F ⬭ DK ⬭	T ⬭ F ⬭ DK ⬭	T ⬭ F ⬭ DK ⬭	T ⬭ F ⬭ DK ⬭
30	T ⬭ F ⬭ DK ⬭	T ⬭ F ⬭ DK ⬭	T ⬭ F ⬭ DK ⬭	T ⬭ F ⬭ DK ⬭	T ⬭ F ⬭ DK ⬭

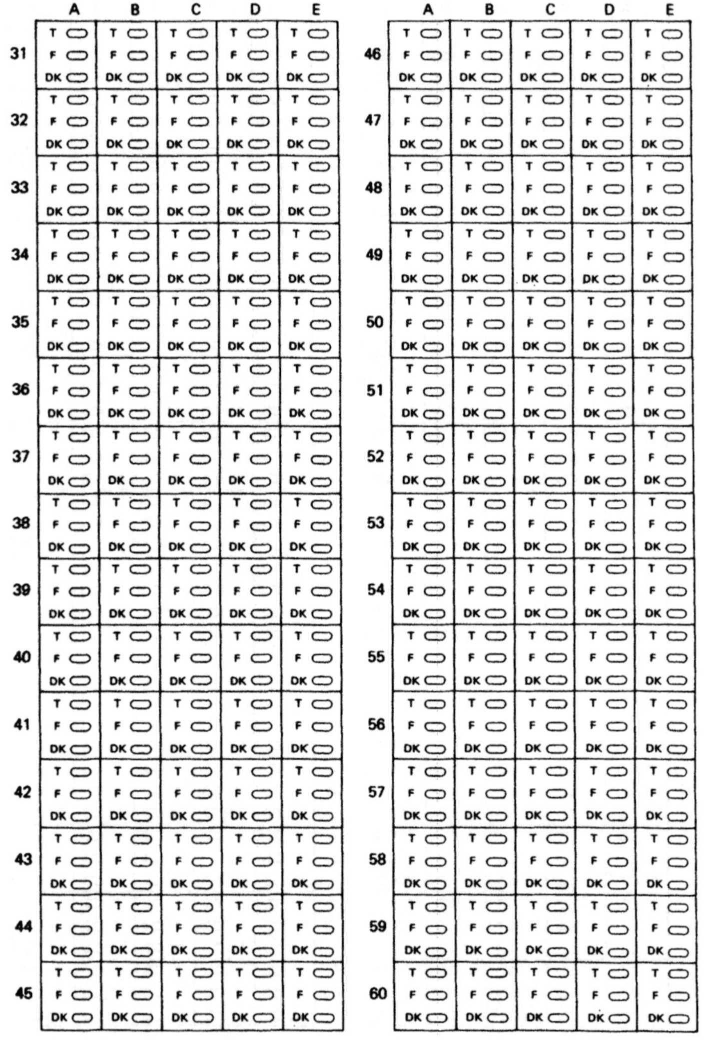

	A	B	C	D	E
31	T F DK	T F DK	T F DK	T F DK	T F DK
32	T F DK	T F DK	T F DK	T F DK	T F DK
33	T F DK	T F DK	T F DK	T F DK	T F DK
34	T F DK	T F DK	T F DK	T F DK	T F DK
35	T F DK	T F DK	T F DK	T F DK	T F DK
36	T F DK	T F DK	T F DK	T F DK	T F DK
37	T F DK	T F DK	T F DK	T F DK	T F DK
38	T F DK	T F DK	T F DK	T F DK	T F DK
39	T F DK	T F DK	T F DK	T F DK	T F DK
40	T F DK	T F DK	T F DK	T F DK	T F DK
41	T F DK	T F DK	T F DK	T F DK	T F DK
42	T F DK	T F DK	T F DK	T F DK	T F DK
43	T F DK	T F DK	T F DK	T F DK	T F DK
44	T F DK	T F DK	T F DK	T F DK	T F DK
45	T F DK	T F DK	T F DK	T F DK	T F DK

	A	B	C	D	E
46	T F DK	T F DK	T F DK	T F DK	T F DK
47	T F DK	T F DK	T F DK	T F DK	T F DK
48	T F DK	T F DK	T F DK	T F DK	T F DK
49	T F DK	T F DK	T F DK	T F DK	T F DK
50	T F DK	T F DK	T F DK	T F DK	T F DK
51	T F DK	T F DK	T F DK	T F DK	T F DK
52	T F DK	T F DK	T F DK	T F DK	T F DK
53	T F DK	T F DK	T F DK	T F DK	T F DK
54	T F DK	T F DK	T F DK	T F DK	T F DK
55	T F DK	T F DK	T F DK	T F DK	T F DK
56	T F DK	T F DK	T F DK	T F DK	T F DK
57	T F DK	T F DK	T F DK	T F DK	T F DK
58	T F DK	T F DK	T F DK	T F DK	T F DK
59	T F DK	T F DK	T F DK	T F DK	T F DK
60	T F DK	T F DK	T F DK	T F DK	T F DK

Q.3.1 Absolute or relative contra-indications to thrombolytic therapy include:

a. Aortic dissection
b. Previous duodenal ulceration
c. Ulcerative colitis
d. Syndrome X
e. Contraceptive pill

Q.3.2 In a patient with a low cardiac output and a low pulmonary capillary wedge pressure, which of the following therapies is indicated:

a. Diuretics
b. Afterload reduction
c. Preload reduction
d. Intravenous fluids
e. Positive inotropes

Q.3.3 Low HDL-cholesterol levels are associated with:

a. Regular exercise
b. Oestrogen therapy
c. Phenytoin therapy
d. Beta blockade
e. Cigarette smoking

Q.3.4 A soft first heart sound is characteristically found in:

a. Pericardial effusion
b. Left ventricular failure
c. Mitral stenosis
d. Complete heart block
e. Wolff–Parkinson–White syndrome

Q.3.5 Which of the following are recognised causes of gastrointestinal blood loss:

a. Pulmonary haemosiderosis
b. Polycythaemia rubra vera
c. Behçet's syndrome
d. Systemic sclerosis
e. Ehlers–Danlos syndrome

Q.3.6 Liver transplantation may be indicated in:

a. Biliary sepsis
b. Fulminant Budd-Chiari syndrome
c. Primary biliary cirrhosis
d. Hepatic metastases
e. Chronic active hepatitis

Q.3.7 In primary biliary cirrhosis:

a. Hypothyroidism is an association
b. There is a high copper concentration in the liver
c. Pruritus usually responds to antihistamine therapy
d. Azathioprine is ineffective
e. There is an association with systemic sclerosis

Q.3.8 Which of the following are purgatives:

a. Aloe
b. Jalap
c. Cascara
d. Frangula
e. Rhubarb

Q.3.9 Non-steroidal anti-inflammatory drugs:

a. Are implicated in 25% of suspected adverse reactions reported to the CSM
b. Are better tolerated in the elderly
c. May cause hypertension
d. May provoke bronchospasm
e. Rarely cause rashes

Q.3.10 Recognised features of sudden discontinuation of prolonged high dose systemic steroid therapy include:

a. Arterial hypotension
b. Hypernatraemia
c. Hypokalaemia
d. Depression
e. Avascular necrosis of the femoral head

Q.3.11 Colloidal bismuth:

a. Eradicates *Helicobacter pylorii* in all cases of peptic ulceration
b. Lightens the stool
c. Darkens the tongue
d. Can cause encephalopathy
e. Affects prostaglandin synthesis

Q.3.12 A crude mortality rate is so called because it:

a. Is not statistically significant
b. Is based on figures from clinical audits
c. Requires later refinement
d. Ignores the age distribution of the population
e. Refers to the rate per unit of area rather than unit of population

Q.3.13 Benign monoclonal gammopathy is associated with:

a. Amyloidosis
b. Gradual increase in paraprotein levels
c. Plasmacytoma
d. Immune paresis
e. Heavy chain disease

Q.3.14 The Wiskott-Aldrich syndrome:

a. Is an autosomal dominant disorder
b. Is associated with thrombocytosis
c. Is associated with eczema
d. Is associated with nephropathy
e. May be complicated by lymphoma

Q.3.15 Polycythaemia may be associated with:

a. Sezary syndrome
b. *Pneumocystis carinii* pneumonia
c. Bronchioalveolar cell carcinoma
d. Ovarian carcinoma
e. Hepatoma

Q.3.16 Which of the following are recognised causes of folate deficiency:

a. Veganism
b. Fish tapeworms
c. Nitrous oxide
d. Zollinger-Ellison syndrome
e. Pernicious anaemia

Q.3.17 Which of the following treatments may be considered for severe bullous emphysema:

a. Radiotherapy
b. Lung transplantation
c. Medical pleurodesis
d. Monaldi procedure
e. Domiciliary oxygen

Q.3.18 Recognised causes of coin-shaped shadows on chest X-ray include:

a. Pneumoconiosis
b. Aspergilloma
c. Rheumatoid arthritis
d. Fibrosing alveolitis
e. Encysted pleural effusion

Q.3.19 Atypical pneumonia is suggested by:

a. Expectoration of purulent sputum
b. Disproportionately severe clinical signs on auscultation compared with chest radiograph
c. Pleuritic chest pain
d. Tachypnoea accompanied by diarrhoea and proteinuria
e. A history of contact with poultry

Q.3.20 Recognised features of combined sodium and water depletion include:

a. Excessive sweating
b. Tetany
c. Postural hypotension
d. Bradycardia
e. Reduced glomerular filtration rate

Q.3.21 Which of the following are recognised to cause tetany:

a. Persistent vomiting
b. Parathyroid adenoma
c. Cri du chat syndrome
d. Protracted topical steroid treatment
e. Malabsorption

Q.3.22 Abdominal pain is a recognised finding in children with:

a. Diabetic ketoacidosis
b. Idiopathic thrombocytopenia
c. Nephrotic syndrome
d. Sickle cell disease
e. Threadworms

Q.3.23 Which of the following are correctly associated:

a. Vitamin D deficiency : muscle weakness
b. Folate deficiency : pregnancy
c. Vitamin C deficiency : subperiosteal haemorrhages
d. Vitamin A deficiency : Wernicke's encephalopathy
e. Thiamine deficiency : peripheral neuropathy

Q.3.24 The pain of:

a. Carpal tunnel syndrome is confined to the hand and wrist
b. Claudication improves when the limb is elevated
c. Pancreatic carcinoma is worsened by sitting
d. Pericarditis is made worse by turning over in bed
e. Myocardial infarction can be felt in the jaw exclusively

Q.3.25 A raised P_aCO_2 is characteristic of:

a. Cor pulmonale
b. Pulmonary embolism
c. Moderately severe asthma
d. Early left ventricular failure
e. Late chronic renal failure

Q.3.26 **Which of the following are recognised features of polycythaemia rubra vera:**

a. Splenomegaly
b. Leucopenia
c. Finger clubbing
d. Arterial hypoxaemia
e. Increased platelet count

Q.3.27 **Oral lesions are commonly seen in:**

a. Measles
b. Rubella
c. Psoriasis
d. Addison's disease
e. Glandular fever

Q.3.28 **Which of the following physical signs are associated with the corresponding conditions:**

a. Jaundice : tricuspid incompetence
b. Palpable spleen : infectious mononucleosis
c. Erythema nodosum : ulcerative colitis
d. Osler's nodes : osteoarthritis
e. Palpable purpura : thrombocytopenia

Q.3.29 **Hypouricaemia is recognised to result from:**

a. Allopurinol overdose
b. Pyrazinamide
c. Carcinomatosis
d. Distal renal tubular disease
e. Aspirin

Q.3.30 **Features of Tangier disease include:**

a. Elevated high density lipoprotein levels
b. Neuropathy
c. Splenomegaly
d. Decreased serum concentration of Apolipoprotein B
e. Orange tonsils

Q.3.31 The nephrotic syndrome:

a. Is associated with a raised serum cholesterol
b. May be caused by pyelonephritis
c. Is associated with heavy proteinuria
d. Is characterised by a low serum albumin concentration
e. Responds well to gold

Q.3.32 Acute renal tubular necrosis is characterised by:

a. Microscopic haematuria
b. A urine/plasma osmolality ratio of 3
c. Oliguria
d. Hypercalcaemia
e. Anaemia

Q.3.33 Which of these gaits and diseases is correctly associated:

a. Festinating – tabes dorsalis
b. Waddling – myopathy
c. Truncal ataxia – Parkinsonism
d. High stepping – Charcot–Marie–Tooth
e. Scissors – spasticity

Q.3.34 Recognised features of raised intracranial pressure include:

a. Vomiting
b. Sixth cranial nerve palsy
c. Tachycardia
d. Enlarged macula
e. Hemicranial headache

Q.3.35 Dementia is characteristically caused by:

a. A manic depressive psychosis
b. Hypothyroidism
c. Amphetamine addiction
d. Normal pressure hydrocephalus
e. Vitamin B12 deficiency

Q.3.36 The following are associated with thrombocytopenia:

a. Alcohol
b. Haemangioma
c. Polycythaemia rubra vera
d. Haemolytic–uraemic syndrome
e. Post splenectomy

Q.3.37 Intracranial haemorrhage:

a. Can be a complication of subacute bacterial endocarditis
b. Is invariably fatal
c. May present with a spastic paraparesis
d. May follow sexual intercourse
e. Causes bradycardia and hypotension

Q.3.38 When the central retinal vein becomes occluded:

a. Visual loss occurs rapidly
b. Glaucoma is an uncommon complication
c. The patient may have had uncontrolled hypertension
d. Neovascularisation of the retina improves the prognosis
e. Hyperlipidaemia should be suspected

Q.3.39 Cutaneous hyperpigmentation is a feature of:

a. Primary failure of cortisol secretion
b. Chronic renal failure
c. Haemochromatosis
d. Systemic lupus erythematosus
e. Hypopituitarism

Q.3.40 Recognised features of thyrotoxicosis include:

a. Liver palms
b. Pruritus
c. Diarrhoea
d. Atrial fibrillation
e. Proximal myopathy

Q.3.41 Which of the following are recognised causes of methaemoglobinaemia:

a. Phosphorous sesquisulphide
b. Mercaptobenzimidazole
c. Trimethylolpropane triacrylate
d. Ethylene thiourea
e. Pentachlorothiophenol

Q.3.42 Infection with human papilloma virus is recognised to cause

a. Adenoma sebaceum
b. Epidermodysplasia verruciformis
c. Molluscum contagiosum
d. Dementia
e. Myrmeccia

Q.3.43 Cervical lymphadenopathy is a recognised finding in:

a. Histiocytic medullary reticulosis
b. Castleman's disease
c. Ménétrièr's disease
d. Urticaria pigmentosa
e. Osler-Weber-Rendu disease

Q.3.44 Which of the following are characteristic of hepatitis A infection:

a. Arthropathy
b. Smooth muscle antibodies in the serum
c. Raised serum aspartate transaminase
d. Bilirubin in the urine
e. Leucocytosis

Q.3.45 Complications of measles include:

a. Orchitis
b. Bronchopneumonia
c. Encephalitis
d. Otitis media
e. Pancreatitis

Q.3.46 Which of the following maternal infections are recognised causes of mental subnormality in a baby:

a. Toxocariasis
b. Hepatitis A
c. *Pneumocystis carinii*
d. Cytomegalovirus infection
e. Toxoplasmosis

Q.3.47 Diabetes mellitus characteristically predisposes to the development of:

a. Otosclerosis
b. Simple glaucoma
c. Intermittent claudication
d. Chronic exocrine pancreatic insufficiency
e. Interstitial keratitis

Q.3.48 Recognised manifestations of acromegaly include:

a. Finger clubbing
b. Cardiomyopathy
c. Deafness
d. Impaired glucose tolerance
e. Dry skin

Q.3.49 Which of the following features would suggest a diagnosis of osteomalacia in an Asian immigrant:

a. Generalised body pain
b. Pruritus
c. Difficulty rising from a chair
d. Polyuria and polydipsia
e. Genu valgus

Q.3.50 Recognised consequences of androgen deficiency include:

a. Premature epiphyseal closure
b. Rugosity of scrotum
c. High pitched voice
d. Hypopituitarism
e. Galactorrhoea

Q.3.51 Recognised side effects of the combined oral contraceptive pill include:

a. Skin pigmentation
b. Hepatoma
c. Cervical erosion
d. Hyperlipidaemia
e. Impaired glucose tolerance

Q.3.52 Luteinising hormone:

a. Is released from the anterior pituitary
b. Stimulates testosterone production from the Leydig cells of the testis
c. Induces ovulation
d. Stimulates the Sertoli cells of the testis to produce spermatozoa
e. Stimulates ovarian oestrogen production

Q.3.53 Recognised causes of hypercalcaemia include:

a. Phosphate administration
b. Diphosphonate therapy
c. Acute pancreatitis
d. Hypomagnesia
e. Vitamin D resistance

Q.3.54 Features of the carcinoid syndrome include:

a. Pruritic wheals
b. Hypotension
c. Pellagra-like rash
d. Mesenteric fibrosis
e. Arthopathy

Q.3.55 Which of the following neoplasms may exhibit hormonal dependence:

a. Wilm's tumour
b. Hepatoma
c. Medullary carcinoma of thyroid
d. Pancreatic carcinoma
e. Clear cell carcinoma of vagina

Q.3.56 Angioid streaks on the retina are recognised to occur in:

a. Pseudoxanthoma elasticum
b. Acromegaly
c. Sickle cell anaemia
d. Paget's disease
e. Ehlers–Danlos syndrome

Q.3.57 Keratitis is a recognised feature of:

a. Herpes simplex infection
b. Glaucoma
c. Exophthalmos
d. Rosacea
e. Acanthamoeba infection

Q.3.58 Fragile X syndrome is associated with:

a. Large testes
b. Mental handicap
c. Autosomal inheritance
d. Response to folate treatment
e. Autism

Q.3.59 The following lesions characteristically blanch with pressure on diascopy:

a. Angiokeratoma in Fabry's disease
b. Campbell de Morgan spots
c. Uraemic thrombocytopaenic purpura
d. Telangiectasia in Osler-Weber-Rendu disease
e. Atrophie blanche

Q.3.60 Carotenaemia may occur in:

a. Hypothyroidism
b. Porphyria
c. Diabetes mellitus
d. Hyperlipidaemia
e. Gout

Examination 4

All parts of every question must be answered *True* or *False* or *Don't Know* by filling in the box provided. Failure to do so will result in rejection of the answer sheet

EXAMINATION NO.
4

SURNAME

[ ]

INITIALS

[ ]

Please use 2B PENCIL only. Rub out all errors thoroughly.
Mark lozenges like ⬬ NOT like this ⊄ ⊄ ⊄

T ⬭ = TRUE   F ⬭ = FALSE   DK ⬭ = DON'T KNOW

	A	B	C	D	E
1	T ⬭ F ⬭ DK ⬭	T ⬭ F ⬭ DK ⬭	T ⬭ F ⬭ DK ⬭	T ⬭ F ⬭ DK ⬭	T ⬭ F ⬭ DK ⬭
2	T ⬭ F ⬭ DK ⬭	T ⬭ F ⬭ DK ⬭	T ⬭ F ⬭ DK ⬭	T ⬭ F ⬭ DK ⬭	T ⬭ F ⬭ DK ⬭
3	T ⬭ F ⬭ DK ⬭	T ⬭ F ⬭ DK ⬭	T ⬭ F ⬭ DK ⬭	T ⬭ F ⬭ DK ⬭	T ⬭ F ⬭ DK ⬭
4	T ⬭ F ⬭ DK ⬭	T ⬭ F ⬭ DK ⬭	T ⬭ F ⬭ DK ⬭	T ⬭ F ⬭ DK ⬭	T ⬭ F ⬭ DK ⬭
5	T ⬭ F ⬭ DK ⬭	T ⬭ F ⬭ DK ⬭	T ⬭ F ⬭ DK ⬭	T ⬭ F ⬭ DK ⬭	T ⬭ F ⬭ DK ⬭
6	T ⬭ F ⬭ DK ⬭	T ⬭ F ⬭ DK ⬭	T ⬭ F ⬭ DK ⬭	T ⬭ F ⬭ DK ⬭	T ⬭ F ⬭ DK ⬭
7	T ⬭ F ⬭ DK ⬭	T ⬭ F ⬭ DK ⬭	T ⬭ F ⬭ DK ⬭	T ⬭ F ⬭ DK ⬭	T ⬭ F ⬭ DK ⬭
8	T ⬭ F ⬭ DK ⬭	T ⬭ F ⬭ DK ⬭	T ⬭ F ⬭ DK ⬭	T ⬭ F ⬭ DK ⬭	T ⬭ F ⬭ DK ⬭
9	T ⬭ F ⬭ DK ⬭	T ⬭ F ⬭ DK ⬭	T ⬭ F ⬭ DK ⬭	T ⬭ F ⬭ DK ⬭	T ⬭ F ⬭ DK ⬭
10	T ⬭ F ⬭ DK ⬭	T ⬭ F ⬭ DK ⬭	T ⬭ F ⬭ DK ⬭	T ⬭ F ⬭ DK ⬭	T ⬭ F ⬭ DK ⬭
11	T ⬭ F ⬭ DK ⬭	T ⬭ F ⬭ DK ⬭	T ⬭ F ⬭ DK ⬭	T ⬭ F ⬭ DK ⬭	T ⬭ F ⬭ DK ⬭
12	T ⬭ F ⬭ DK ⬭	T ⬭ F ⬭ DK ⬭	T ⬭ F ⬭ DK ⬭	T ⬭ F ⬭ DK ⬭	T ⬭ F ⬭ DK ⬭
13	T ⬭ F ⬭ DK ⬭	T ⬭ F ⬭ DK ⬭	T ⬭ F ⬭ DK ⬭	T ⬭ F ⬭ DK ⬭	T ⬭ F ⬭ DK ⬭
14	T ⬭ F ⬭ DK ⬭	T ⬭ F ⬭ DK ⬭	T ⬭ F ⬭ DK ⬭	T ⬭ F ⬭ DK ⬭	T ⬭ F ⬭ DK ⬭
15	T ⬭ F ⬭ DK ⬭	T ⬭ F ⬭ DK ⬭	T ⬭ F ⬭ DK ⬭	T ⬭ F ⬭ DK ⬭	T ⬭ F ⬭ DK ⬭
16	T ⬭ F ⬭ DK ⬭	T ⬭ F ⬭ DK ⬭	T ⬭ F ⬭ DK ⬭	T ⬭ F ⬭ DK ⬭	T ⬭ F ⬭ DK ⬭
17	T ⬭ F ⬭ DK ⬭	T ⬭ F ⬭ DK ⬭	T ⬭ F ⬭ DK ⬭	T ⬭ F ⬭ DK ⬭	T ⬭ F ⬭ DK ⬭
18	T ⬭ F ⬭ DK ⬭	T ⬭ F ⬭ DK ⬭	T ⬭ F ⬭ DK ⬭	T ⬭ F ⬭ DK ⬭	T ⬭ F ⬭ DK ⬭
19	T ⬭ F ⬭ DK ⬭	T ⬭ F ⬭ DK ⬭	T ⬭ F ⬭ DK ⬭	T ⬭ F ⬭ DK ⬭	T ⬭ F ⬭ DK ⬭
20	T ⬭ F ⬭ DK ⬭	T ⬭ F ⬭ DK ⬭	T ⬭ F ⬭ DK ⬭	T ⬭ F ⬭ DK ⬭	T ⬭ F ⬭ DK ⬭
21	T ⬭ F ⬭ DK ⬭	T ⬭ F ⬭ DK ⬭	T ⬭ F ⬭ DK ⬭	T ⬭ F ⬭ DK ⬭	T ⬭ F ⬭ DK ⬭
22	T ⬭ F ⬭ DK ⬭	T ⬭ F ⬭ DK ⬭	T ⬭ F ⬭ DK ⬭	T ⬭ F ⬭ DK ⬭	T ⬭ F ⬭ DK ⬭
23	T ⬭ F ⬭ DK ⬭	T ⬭ F ⬭ DK ⬭	T ⬭ F ⬭ DK ⬭	T ⬭ F ⬭ DK ⬭	T ⬭ F ⬭ DK ⬭
24	T ⬭ F ⬭ DK ⬭	T ⬭ F ⬭ DK ⬭	T ⬭ F ⬭ DK ⬭	T ⬭ F ⬭ DK ⬭	T ⬭ F ⬭ DK ⬭
25	T ⬭ F ⬭ DK ⬭	T ⬭ F ⬭ DK ⬭	T ⬭ F ⬭ DK ⬭	T ⬭ F ⬭ DK ⬭	T ⬭ F ⬭ DK ⬭
26	T ⬭ F ⬭ DK ⬭	T ⬭ F ⬭ DK ⬭	T ⬭ F ⬭ DK ⬭	T ⬭ F ⬭ DK ⬭	T ⬭ F ⬭ DK ⬭
27	T ⬭ F ⬭ DK ⬭	T ⬭ F ⬭ DK ⬭	T ⬭ F ⬭ DK ⬭	T ⬭ F ⬭ DK ⬭	T ⬭ F ⬭ DK ⬭
28	T ⬭ F ⬭ DK ⬭	T ⬭ F ⬭ DK ⬭	T ⬭ F ⬭ DK ⬭	T ⬭ F ⬭ DK ⬭	T ⬭ F ⬭ DK ⬭
29	T ⬭ F ⬭ DK ⬭	T ⬭ F ⬭ DK ⬭	T ⬭ F ⬭ DK ⬭	T ⬭ F ⬭ DK ⬭	T ⬭ F ⬭ DK ⬭
30	T ⬭ F ⬭ DK ⬭	T ⬭ F ⬭ DK ⬭	T ⬭ F ⬭ DK ⬭	T ⬭ F ⬭ DK ⬭	T ⬭ F ⬭ DK ⬭

	A	B	C	D	E
31	T ⬭ F ⬭ DK ⬭	T ⬭ F ⬭ DK ⬭	T ⬭ F ⬭ DK ⬭	T ⬭ F ⬭ DK ⬭	T ⬭ F ⬭ DK ⬭
32	T ⬭ F ⬭ DK ⬭	T ⬭ F ⬭ DK ⬭	T ⬭ F ⬭ DK ⬭	T ⬭ F ⬭ DK ⬭	T ⬭ F ⬭ DK ⬭
33	T ⬭ F ⬭ DK ⬭	T ⬭ F ⬭ DK ⬭	T ⬭ F ⬭ DK ⬭	T ⬭ F ⬭ DK ⬭	T ⬭ F ⬭ DK ⬭
34	T ⬭ F ⬭ DK ⬭	T ⬭ F ⬭ DK ⬭	T ⬭ F ⬭ DK ⬭	T ⬭ F ⬭ DK ⬭	T ⬭ F ⬭ DK ⬭
35	T ⬭ F ⬭ DK ⬭	T ⬭ F ⬭ DK ⬭	T ⬭ F ⬭ DK ⬭	T ⬭ F ⬭ DK ⬭	T ⬭ F ⬭ DK ⬭
36	T ⬭ F ⬭ DK ⬭	T ⬭ F ⬭ DK ⬭	T ⬭ F ⬭ DK ⬭	T ⬭ F ⬭ DK ⬭	T ⬭ F ⬭ DK ⬭
37	T ⬭ F ⬭ DK ⬭	T ⬭ F ⬭ DK ⬭	T ⬭ F ⬭ DK ⬭	T ⬭ F ⬭ DK ⬭	T ⬭ F ⬭ DK ⬭
38	T ⬭ F ⬭ DK ⬭	T ⬭ F ⬭ DK ⬭	T ⬭ F ⬭ DK ⬭	T ⬭ F ⬭ DK ⬭	T ⬭ F ⬭ DK ⬭
39	T ⬭ F ⬭ DK ⬭	T ⬭ F ⬭ DK ⬭	T ⬭ F ⬭ DK ⬭	T ⬭ F ⬭ DK ⬭	T ⬭ F ⬭ DK ⬭
40	T ⬭ F ⬭ DK ⬭	T ⬭ F ⬭ DK ⬭	T ⬭ F ⬭ DK ⬭	T ⬭ F ⬭ DK ⬭	T ⬭ F ⬭ DK ⬭
41	T ⬭ F ⬭ DK ⬭	T ⬭ F ⬭ DK ⬭	T ⬭ F ⬭ DK ⬭	T ⬭ F ⬭ DK ⬭	T ⬭ F ⬭ DK ⬭
42	T ⬭ F ⬭ DK ⬭	T ⬭ F ⬭ DK ⬭	T ⬭ F ⬭ DK ⬭	T ⬭ F ⬭ DK ⬭	T ⬭ F ⬭ DK ⬭
43	T ⬭ F ⬭ DK ⬭	T ⬭ F ⬭ DK ⬭	T ⬭ F ⬭ DK ⬭	T ⬭ F ⬭ DK ⬭	T ⬭ F ⬭ DK ⬭
44	T ⬭ F ⬭ DK ⬭	T ⬭ F ⬭ DK ⬭	T ⬭ F ⬭ DK ⬭	T ⬭ F ⬭ DK ⬭	T ⬭ F ⬭ DK ⬭
45	T ⬭ F ⬭ DK ⬭	T ⬭ F ⬭ DK ⬭	T ⬭ F ⬭ DK ⬭	T ⬭ F ⬭ DK ⬭	T ⬭ F ⬭ DK ⬭

	A	B	C	D	E
46	T ⬭ F ⬭ DK ⬭	T ⬭ F ⬭ DK ⬭	T ⬭ F ⬭ DK ⬭	T ⬭ F ⬭ DK ⬭	T ⬭ F ⬭ DK ⬭
47	T ⬭ F ⬭ DK ⬭	T ⬭ F ⬭ DK ⬭	T ⬭ F ⬭ DK ⬭	T ⬭ F ⬭ DK ⬭	T ⬭ F ⬭ DK ⬭
48	T ⬭ F ⬭ DK ⬭	T ⬭ F ⬭ DK ⬭	T ⬭ F ⬭ DK ⬭	T ⬭ F ⬭ DK ⬭	T ⬭ F ⬭ DK ⬭
49	T ⬭ F ⬭ DK ⬭	T ⬭ F ⬭ DK ⬭	T ⬭ F ⬭ DK ⬭	T ⬭ F ⬭ DK ⬭	T ⬭ F ⬭ DK ⬭
50	T ⬭ F ⬭ DK ⬭	T ⬭ F ⬭ DK ⬭	T ⬭ F ⬭ DK ⬭	T ⬭ F ⬭ DK ⬭	T ⬭ F ⬭ DK ⬭
51	T ⬭ F ⬭ DK ⬭	T ⬭ F ⬭ DK ⬭	T ⬭ F ⬭ DK ⬭	T ⬭ F ⬭ DK ⬭	T ⬭ F ⬭ DK ⬭
52	T ⬭ F ⬭ DK ⬭	T ⬭ F ⬭ DK ⬭	T ⬭ F ⬭ DK ⬭	T ⬭ F ⬭ DK ⬭	T ⬭ F ⬭ DK ⬭
53	T ⬭ F ⬭ DK ⬭	T ⬭ F ⬭ DK ⬭	T ⬭ F ⬭ DK ⬭	T ⬭ F ⬭ DK ⬭	T ⬭ F ⬭ DK ⬭
54	T ⬭ F ⬭ DK ⬭	T ⬭ F ⬭ DK ⬭	T ⬭ F ⬭ DK ⬭	T ⬭ F ⬭ DK ⬭	T ⬭ F ⬭ DK ⬭
55	T ⬭ F ⬭ DK ⬭	T ⬭ F ⬭ DK ⬭	T ⬭ F ⬭ DK ⬭	T ⬭ F ⬭ DK ⬭	T ⬭ F ⬭ DK ⬭
56	T ⬭ F ⬭ DK ⬭	T ⬭ F ⬭ DK ⬭	T ⬭ F ⬭ DK ⬭	T ⬭ F ⬭ DK ⬭	T ⬭ F ⬭ DK ⬭
57	T ⬭ F ⬭ DK ⬭	T ⬭ F ⬭ DK ⬭	T ⬭ F ⬭ DK ⬭	T ⬭ F ⬭ DK ⬭	T ⬭ F ⬭ DK ⬭
58	T ⬭ F ⬭ DK ⬭	T ⬭ F ⬭ DK ⬭	T ⬭ F ⬭ DK ⬭	T ⬭ F ⬭ DK ⬭	T ⬭ F ⬭ DK ⬭
59	T ⬭ F ⬭ DK ⬭	T ⬭ F ⬭ DK ⬭	T ⬭ F ⬭ DK ⬭	T ⬭ F ⬭ DK ⬭	T ⬭ F ⬭ DK ⬭
60	T ⬭ F ⬭ DK ⬭	T ⬭ F ⬭ DK ⬭	T ⬭ F ⬭ DK ⬭	T ⬭ F ⬭ DK ⬭	T ⬭ F ⬭ DK ⬭

Q.4.1 Paradoxical splitting of the second heart occurs in:

a. Atrial septal defect
b. Calcium antagonist therapy
c. Patent ductus arteriosus
d. Hypertrophic obstructive cardiomyopathy
e. Anomalous pulmonary venous drainage

Q.4.2 Which of these are risk factors for ischaemic heart disease:

a. Coal mining
b. Hypertension
c. Hypercholesterolaemia
d. Diabetes mellitus
e. Asthma

Q.4.3 There is an rapid 'y' descent of the JVP in:

a. Acute pulmonary embolism
b. Aortic stenosis
c. Atrial fibrillation
d. Constrictive pericarditis
e. Digoxin toxicity

Q.4.4 Indications of severe aortic stenosis include:

a. Pulse pressure of 50mm Hg
b. Third heart sound
c. Austin Flint murmur
d. Left ventricular ejection fraction of 50%
e. Giant 'a' wave

Q.4.5 Cholecystokinin:

a. Stimulates gastric secretion
b. Releases pancreatic enzymes
c. Reduces gastric emptying
d. Increases lower oesophageal sphincter tone
e. Releases pancreatic bicarbonate

Q.4.6 Recognised indications for emergency surgery in ulcerative colitis include:

a. Toxic dilatation of the colon
b. Persistent active disease
c. Premalignant mucosal changes
d. Perforation
e. Haemorrhage

Q.4.7 The differential diagnosis of hepatosplenomegaly includes:

a. Constrictive pericarditis
b. Alcoholic hepatitis
c. Amyloidosis
d. Mastocytosis
e. Sarcoidosis

Q.4.8 Jejunal ulceration is a recognised feature of:

a. Crohn's disease
b. Lymphoma
c. Tuberculosis
d. Potassium tablets
e. Polyarteritis nodosa

Q.4.9 Which of the following drugs are recognised to interfere with neuromuscular transmission:

a. Phenytoin
b. Gentamicin
c. Curare
d. Lithium
e. Aspirin

Q.4.10 Which of the following cytotoxic drugs are cycle specific and phase specific:

a. Cyclophosphamide
b. Bleomycin
c. Doxorubicin
d. Vincristine
e. Busulphan

Q.4.11 Recognised consequences of high-dose oral corticosteroid therapy include:

a. Acute psychosis
b. Elevated alkakine phosphatase
c. Cataracts
d. Osteomalacia
e. Growth retardation in children

Q.4.12 Complications of digoxin include:

a. Hypocalcaemia
b. Renal failure
c. Sinus bradycardia
d. Ventricular tachycardia
e. Anorexia

Q.4.13 Haemolytic anaemia is recognised to occur in:

a. Infectious mononucleosis
b. Mycoplasma pneumonia
c. Yersinia pestis
d. Falciparum malaria
e. Actinomycosis

Q.4.14 Acute haemolytic anaemia is characterised by:

a. Pruritus
b. Bone marrow depression
c. Leg ulcers
d. Reticulocytosis
e. Bilirubin in the urine

Q.4.15 The following may be early clinical manifestations of primary biliary cirrhosis:

a. Dementia
b. Ascites
c. Campbell de Morgan spots
d. Liver spots
e. Pruritus

Q.4.16 With gradual progressive unilateral spastic weakness of the leg without other abnormalities the diagnosis may be:

a. Parasagittal meningioma
b. Intracerebral metastasis
c. A cerebrovascular accident
d. Vitamin B complex deficiency
e. Multiple sclerosis

Q.4.17 High dose inhaled corticosteroid therapy is a recognised cause of:

a. Myopathy
b. Osteoporosis
c. Diabetes mellitus
d. Candidiasis
e. Hypertension

Q.4.18 Haemoptysis is a recognised manifestation of:

a. Emphysema
b. Pulmonary aspergilloma
c. Extrinsic allergic alveolitis
d. Bronchial adenoma
e. Mitral stenosis

Q.4.19 Acute epiglottitis is:

a. Usually caused by streptococcal pneumonia in children
b. Associated with laryngeal obstruction
c. Associated with fever and tachycardia
d. Diagnosed by taking a lateral neck x-ray
e. Is very rare over the age of 2 years

Q.4.20 Recognised features of carcinoma of the bronchus include:

a. Hypokalaemic acidosis
b. Hypernatraemia
c. Peripheral neuropathy
d. Hypocalcaemia
e. Hypertrophic pulmonary osteoarthropathy

Q.4.21 Factors associated with time lost from work through sickness in the UK include:

a. Male sex
b. Unskilled occupations
c. Respiratory illnesses
d. Cancer (all forms) rather than musculo-skeletal disorders
e. A gradual increase over the last decade

Q.4.22 Atrial fibrillation is a recognised complication of:

a. Aortic stenosis
b. Carcinoma of the bronchus
c. Tricuspid regurgitation
d. Non-toxic goitre
e. Ischaemic heart disease

Q.4.23 Within 4 hours of a large aspirin overdose:

a. Hyperventilation indicates a metabolic alkalosis
b. A normal state of consciousness is expected
c. Gastric lavage is indicated
d. A forced acid diuresis is indicated
e. Renal damage should be anticipated

Q.4.24 Appropriate treatment of portal-systemic encephalopathy includes:

a. Protein restriction
b. Fructose infusion
c. High dose steroid therapy
d. Lactulose
e. Chlormethiazole

Q.4.25 Patients with severe agoraphobia:

a. Are often also afraid of enclosed spaces
b. Are characteristically of low I.Q.
c. Are usually male
d. Experience episodes of severe depression
e. Avoid travelling

Q.4.26 The prevalence of a disease may be estimated from:

a. The proportion of hospital admissions with that disease
b. The proportion of hospital beds occupied by patients with the disease
c. The proportion of persons with the disease in a random sample of the population
d. The number of new cases occurring each year in a representative general practice of known size
e. The mortality rate from that disease

Q.4.27 Clinical features of chronic renal failure include:

a. Prognathism
b. Cutaneous hyperpigmentation
c. Back-ache
d. Pruritus
e. Anorexia

Q.4.28 The following may be found in normal healthy adults:

a. A palpable right kidney
b. Prominent pulsations of the temporal artery
c. Clubbing of the fingers
d. A palpable spleen
e. A soft parasternal ejection systolic mumur

Q.4.29 Clinically important causes of hypophosphataemia include:

a. Distal renal tubular dysfunction
b. Severe burns
c. Hyperalimentation
d. Insulin therapy of diabetic ketoacidosis
e. Phosphate enemas

Q.4.30 Causes of malabsorption of fat include:

a. Malaria
b. Cholecystectomy
c. Hypervitaminosis A
d. Hypothyroidism
e. Giardiasis

Q.4.31 Recognised causes of high blood pressure include:

a. Cerebral haemorrhage
b. Sodium losing enteropathy
c. Patent ductus arteriosus
d. Adenoma of the zona glomerulosa
e. Renal artery stenosis

Q.4.32 Causes of clubbing include:

a. Crohn's disease
b. Psoriasis
c. Bacterial endocarditis
d. Raynaud's phenomenon
e. Renal osteodystrophy

Q.4.33 Recognised causes of peripheral sensory neuropathy include:

a. Lead poisoning
b. Malaria
c. Herpes zoster
d. Uraemia
e. Alcohol

Q.4.34 Progressive multifocal leucoencephalopathy is associated with:

a. Normal CSF examination
b. Lymphoma
c. Prolonged (> 1 year) survival
d. Flushing
e. Improvement with guanidine

Q.4.35 Recognised associations with the Eaton–Lambert Syndrome include:

a. Hyporeflexia
b. Oculo-bulbar weakness
c. Improvement with guanidine
d. Pretetanic facilitation on EMG
e. Muscle wasting

Q.4.36 An extensor plantar response is a recognised sign in:

a. Lesions of the anterior horn cells
b. Post-ictal states
c. Vitamin B12 deficiency
d. Thiamine deficiency
e. Hyperglycaemic coma

Q.4.37 The following are features of Behçet's disease:

a. Erythema multiforme
b. Recurrent deep venous thrombosis
c. Erythema nodosum
d. Granuloma formation
e. Iritis

Q.4.38 Recognised features of severe depression include:

a. Early morning wakening
b. Agitation
c. Loss of appetite
d. Dementia
e. Hypochondriacal delusions

Q.4.39 The carpal tunnel syndrome:

a. May be associated with pain in the forearm
b. Occurs in systemic sclerosis
c. Is more painful at night
d. Occurs in pregnancy
e. Is associated with wasting of the hypothenar eminence

Q.4.40 The following are paired correctly:

a. Throbbing pulse : cor pulmonale
b. Collapsing pulse : severe anaemia
c. Slowly rising pulse : myxoedema
d. Paradoxical pulse : constrictive pericarditis
e. Bigeminal pulse : digoxin intoxication

Q.4.41 Radiological features of ulcerative colitis include:

a. Distensible rectum
b. Pseudo-polyps
c. Pyoderma gangrenosum
d. Hyperosteophytosis
e. Narrowing of the colonic lumen

Q.4.42 Complications of diabetes mellitus include:

a. Macular oedema
b. Postural hypotension
c. Proteinuria
d. Pruritus
e. Nocturnal diarrhoea

Q.4.43 Haemoptysis is a recognised feature of:

a. Asthma
b. *Pneumocystis carinii* pneumonia
c. Lobar pneumonia
d. Spontaneous pneumothorax
e. Mitral stenosis

Q.4.44 Obesity predisposes to:

a. Muscle weakness
b. Basal cell papillomas
c. Insulin-dependent diabetes mellitus
d. Sleep apnoea
e. Osteoporosis

Q.4.45 Features of cirrhosis include:

a. Bitemporal hemianopia
b. A small liver
c. Splenomegaly
d. Ankle oedema
e. Testicular atrophy

Q.4.46 Features of whooping cough include:

a. Pharyngeal pseudomembrane
b. Bradycardia
c. Hypoxia during coughing spasms
d. Lymphopenia
e. Conjunctival haemorrhages

Q.4.47 Recognised causes of hypoglycaemia:

a. Prolonged starvation
b. Fulminant hepatitis A
c. Ethanol ingestion
d. Carcinoid syndrome
e. Hypopituitarism

Q.4.48 Infective endocarditis:

a. Is a notifiable disease
b. Is rare on prosthetic valves
c. Commonly affects the mitral valve
d. May cause microscopic haematuria
e. Can be excluded if no cardiac murmur is heard

Q.4.49 Grave's disease may cause:

a. Breathlessness
b. Myopathy
c. Pruritus
d. Ophthalmoplegia
e. Weight loss

Q.4.50 Recognised clinical features of the onset of diabetic nephropathy include:

a. Oliguria
b. Decreasing microalbuminuria
c. Increased insulin requirement
d. Increasing glycosuria
e. More frequent hypoglycaemic episodes

Q.4.51 A flat TRH stimulation test is found in:

a. Thyrotoxicosis
b. Hypothalamic disease
c. Primary hypothyroidism
d. Acromegaly
e. Pregnancy

Q.4.52 Which of these hormones are released by stress:

a. ADH
b. TSH
c. LH
d. Insulin
e. Prolactin

Q.4.53 Recognised features of phaeochromocytoma include:

a. Anxiety
b. Glycosuria
c. Chest pain
d. Raynaud's phenomenon
e. Headache

Q.4.54 Recognised features of insulinoma include:

a. Diplopia
b. Grand mal epilepsy
c. Abnormal glucose tolerance test
d. Sweating
e. Bradycardia

Q.4.55 Carbon monoxide poisoning:

a. Causes 10,000 deaths per year in the UK
b. May cause skin necrosis
c. Causes tardive dyskinesia
d. Results in skin pallor more commonly than a cherry red colour
e. Is the main cause of death by poisoning in children

Q.4.56 Which of the following are recognised features of vitiligo:

a. Predisposition to basal cell cancer
b. Prolonged survival in melanoma
c. The Koebner phenomenon
d. An autoimmune response directed against melanocytes
e. Successful treatment by P-UVA

Q.4.57 Splinter haemorrhages are recognised features of:

a. Severe anaemia
b. Trichinosis
c. Leukaemia
d. Systemic lupus erythematosus
e. Meningococcal septicaemia

Q.4.58 Which of the following associations are correct:

a. Mesothelioma and smoking
b. Bladder cancer and analgesic abuse
c. Oesophageal cancer and Plummer–Vinson Syndrome
d. Colorectal cancer and *Clonorchis* infestation
e. Lung cancer and cardiac disease

Q.4.59 Autosomal recessive inheritance is:

a. Often associated with consanguinity
b. Often associated with a specific enzyme defect
c. Responsible for disease in 2.5 per 1000 births in the UK
d. Responsible for sickle cell anaemia
e. Excluded by direct male to male transmission

Q.4.60 Endometriosis:

a. Is commonest in multiparous black women
b. May be due to retrograde menstruation
c. May be found in 20% of all gynaecological laparoscopies
d. Is effectively treated with danazol
e. Often presents with haematuria

Examination 5

All parts of every question must be answered *True* or *False* or *Don't Know* by filling in the box provided. Failure to do so will result in rejection of the answer sheet

EXAMINATION NO.
5

SURNAME

INITIALS

Please use 2B PENCIL only. Rub out all errors thoroughly.
Mark lozenges like ▬ NOT like this ⌀ ⌀ ⌀

T ⬭ = TRUE F ⬭ = FALSE DK ⬭ = DON'T KNOW

	A	B	C	D	E
1	T ⬭ F ⬭ DK ⬭	T ⬭ F ⬭ DK ⬭	T ⬭ F ⬭ DK ⬭	T ⬭ F ⬭ DK ⬭	T ⬭ F ⬭ DK ⬭
2	T ⬭ F ⬭ DK ⬭	T ⬭ F ⬭ DK ⬭	T ⬭ F ⬭ DK ⬭	T ⬭ F ⬭ DK ⬭	T ⬭ F ⬭ DK ⬭
3	T ⬭ F ⬭ DK ⬭	T ⬭ F ⬭ DK ⬭	T ⬭ F ⬭ DK ⬭	T ⬭ F ⬭ DK ⬭	T ⬭ F ⬭ DK ⬭
4	T ⬭ F ⬭ DK ⬭	T ⬭ F ⬭ DK ⬭	T ⬭ F ⬭ DK ⬭	T ⬭ F ⬭ DK ⬭	T ⬭ F ⬭ DK ⬭
5	T ⬭ F ⬭ DK ⬭	T ⬭ F ⬭ DK ⬭	T ⬭ F ⬭ DK ⬭	T ⬭ F ⬭ DK ⬭	T ⬭ F ⬭ DK ⬭
6	T ⬭ F ⬭ DK ⬭	T ⬭ F ⬭ DK ⬭	T ⬭ F ⬭ DK ⬭	T ⬭ F ⬭ DK ⬭	T ⬭ F ⬭ DK ⬭
7	T ⬭ F ⬭ DK ⬭	T ⬭ F ⬭ DK ⬭	T ⬭ F ⬭ DK ⬭	T ⬭ F ⬭ DK ⬭	T ⬭ F ⬭ DK ⬭
8	T ⬭ F ⬭ DK ⬭	T ⬭ F ⬭ DK ⬭	T ⬭ F ⬭ DK ⬭	T ⬭ F ⬭ DK ⬭	T ⬭ F ⬭ DK ⬭
9	T ⬭ F ⬭ DK ⬭	T ⬭ F ⬭ DK ⬭	T ⬭ F ⬭ DK ⬭	T ⬭ F ⬭ DK ⬭	T ⬭ F ⬭ DK ⬭
10	T ⬭ F ⬭ DK ⬭	T ⬭ F ⬭ DK ⬭	T ⬭ F ⬭ DK ⬭	T ⬭ F ⬭ DK ⬭	T ⬭ F ⬭ DK ⬭
11	T ⬭ F ⬭ DK ⬭	T ⬭ F ⬭ DK ⬭	T ⬭ F ⬭ DK ⬭	T ⬭ F ⬭ DK ⬭	T ⬭ F ⬭ DK ⬭
12	T ⬭ F ⬭ DK ⬭	T ⬭ F ⬭ DK ⬭	T ⬭ F ⬭ DK ⬭	T ⬭ F ⬭ DK ⬭	T ⬭ F ⬭ DK ⬭
13	T ⬭ F ⬭ DK ⬭	T ⬭ F ⬭ DK ⬭	T ⬭ F ⬭ DK ⬭	T ⬭ F ⬭ DK ⬭	T ⬭ F ⬭ DK ⬭
14	T ⬭ F ⬭ DK ⬭	T ⬭ F ⬭ DK ⬭	T ⬭ F ⬭ DK ⬭	T ⬭ F ⬭ DK ⬭	T ⬭ F ⬭ DK ⬭
15	T ⬭ F ⬭ DK ⬭	T ⬭ F ⬭ DK ⬭	T ⬭ F ⬭ DK ⬭	T ⬭ F ⬭ DK ⬭	T ⬭ F ⬭ DK ⬭

	A	B	C	D	E
16	T ⬭ F ⬭ DK ⬭	T ⬭ F ⬭ DK ⬭	T ⬭ F ⬭ DK ⬭	T ⬭ F ⬭ DK ⬭	T ⬭ F ⬭ DK ⬭
17	T ⬭ F ⬭ DK ⬭	T ⬭ F ⬭ DK ⬭	T ⬭ F ⬭ DK ⬭	T ⬭ F ⬭ DK ⬭	T ⬭ F ⬭ DK ⬭
18	T ⬭ F ⬭ DK ⬭	T ⬭ F ⬭ DK ⬭	T ⬭ F ⬭ DK ⬭	T ⬭ F ⬭ DK ⬭	T ⬭ F ⬭ DK ⬭
19	T ⬭ F ⬭ DK ⬭	T ⬭ F ⬭ DK ⬭	T ⬭ F ⬭ DK ⬭	T ⬭ F ⬭ DK ⬭	T ⬭ F ⬭ DK ⬭
20	T ⬭ F ⬭ DK ⬭	T ⬭ F ⬭ DK ⬭	T ⬭ F ⬭ DK ⬭	T ⬭ F ⬭ DK ⬭	T ⬭ F ⬭ DK ⬭
21	T ⬭ F ⬭ DK ⬭	T ⬭ F ⬭ DK ⬭	T ⬭ F ⬭ DK ⬭	T ⬭ F ⬭ DK ⬭	T ⬭ F ⬭ DK ⬭
22	T ⬭ F ⬭ DK ⬭	T ⬭ F ⬭ DK ⬭	T ⬭ F ⬭ DK ⬭	T ⬭ F ⬭ DK ⬭	T ⬭ F ⬭ DK ⬭
23	T ⬭ F ⬭ DK ⬭	T ⬭ F ⬭ DK ⬭	T ⬭ F ⬭ DK ⬭	T ⬭ F ⬭ DK ⬭	T ⬭ F ⬭ DK ⬭
24	T ⬭ F ⬭ DK ⬭	T ⬭ F ⬭ DK ⬭	T ⬭ F ⬭ DK ⬭	T ⬭ F ⬭ DK ⬭	T ⬭ F ⬭ DK ⬭
25	T ⬭ F ⬭ DK ⬭	T ⬭ F ⬭ DK ⬭	T ⬭ F ⬭ DK ⬭	T ⬭ F ⬭ DK ⬭	T ⬭ F ⬭ DK ⬭
26	T ⬭ F ⬭ DK ⬭	T ⬭ F ⬭ DK ⬭	T ⬭ F ⬭ DK ⬭	T ⬭ F ⬭ DK ⬭	T ⬭ F ⬭ DK ⬭
27	T ⬭ F ⬭ DK ⬭	T ⬭ F ⬭ DK ⬭	T ⬭ F ⬭ DK ⬭	T ⬭ F ⬭ DK ⬭	T ⬭ F ⬭ DK ⬭
28	T ⬭ F ⬭ DK ⬭	T ⬭ F ⬭ DK ⬭	T ⬭ F ⬭ DK ⬭	T ⬭ F ⬭ DK ⬭	T ⬭ F ⬭ DK ⬭
29	T ⬭ F ⬭ DK ⬭	T ⬭ F ⬭ DK ⬭	T ⬭ F ⬭ DK ⬭	T ⬭ F ⬭ DK ⬭	T ⬭ F ⬭ DK ⬭
30	T ⬭ F ⬭ DK ⬭	T ⬭ F ⬭ DK ⬭	T ⬭ F ⬭ DK ⬭	T ⬭ F ⬭ DK ⬭	T ⬭ F ⬭ DK ⬭

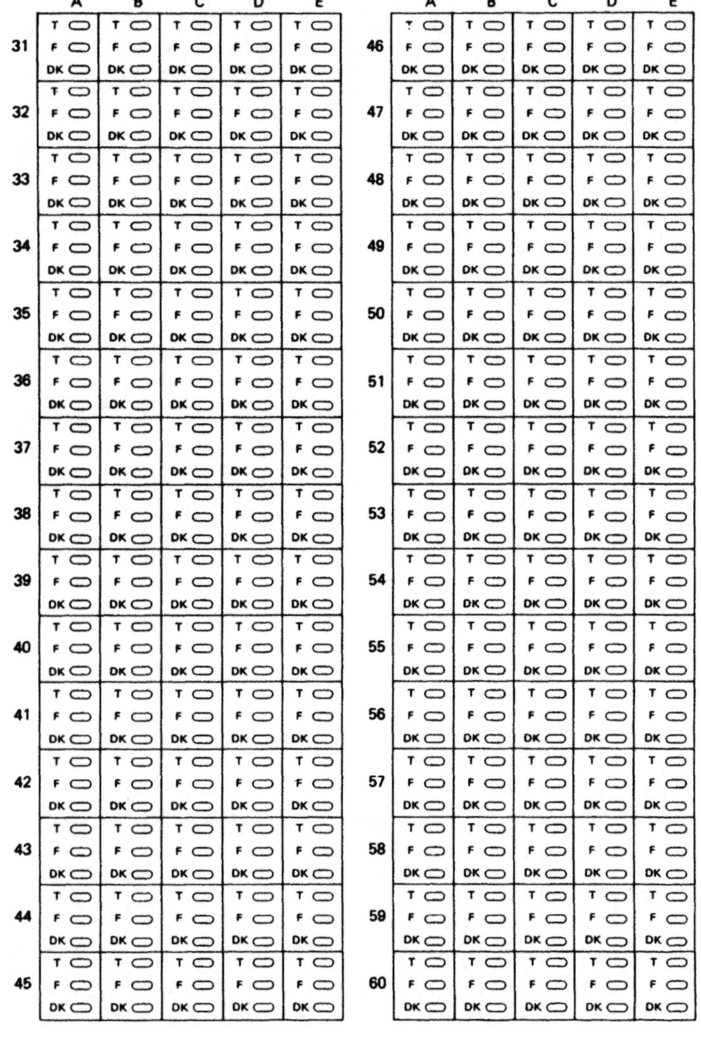

	A	B	C	D	E
31	T F DK	T F DK	T F DK	T F DK	T F DK
32	T F DK	T F DK	T F DK	T F DK	T F DK
33	T F DK	T F DK	T F DK	T F DK	T F DK
34	T F DK	T F DK	T F DK	T F DK	T F DK
35	T F DK	T F DK	T F DK	T F DK	T F DK
36	T F DK	T F DK	T F DK	T F DK	T F DK
37	T F DK	T F DK	T F DK	T F DK	T F DK
38	T F DK	T F DK	T F DK	T F DK	T F DK
39	T F DK	T F DK	T F DK	T F DK	T F DK
40	T F DK	T F DK	T F DK	T F DK	T F DK
41	T F DK	T F DK	T F DK	T F DK	T F DK
42	T F DK	T F DK	T F DK	T F DK	T F DK
43	T F DK	T F DK	T F DK	T F DK	T F DK
44	T F DK	T F DK	T F DK	T F DK	T F DK
45	T F DK	T F DK	T F DK	T F DK	T F DK

	A	B	C	D	E
46	T F DK	T F DK	T F DK	T F DK	T F DK
47	T F DK	T F DK	T F DK	T F DK	T F DK
48	T F DK	T F DK	T F DK	T F DK	T F DK
49	T F DK	T F DK	T F DK	T F DK	T F DK
50	T F DK	T F DK	T F DK	T F DK	T F DK
51	T F DK	T F DK	T F DK	T F DK	T F DK
52	T F DK	T F DK	T F DK	T F DK	T F DK
53	T F DK	T F DK	T F DK	T F DK	T F DK
54	T F DK	T F DK	T F DK	T F DK	T F DK
55	T F DK	T F DK	T F DK	T F DK	T F DK
56	T F DK	T F DK	T F DK	T F DK	T F DK
57	T F DK	T F DK	T F DK	T F DK	T F DK
58	T F DK	T F DK	T F DK	T F DK	T F DK
59	T F DK	T F DK	T F DK	T F DK	T F DK
60	T F DK	T F DK	T F DK	T F DK	T F DK

Q.5.1 Which of the following are recognised as possible complications in coronary angioplasty:

a. Cardiac tamponade
b. Cerebral embolism
c. Ventricular dysrhythmias
d. Coronary dissection
e. Femoral artery occlusion

Q.5.2 Cardiac preload is reduced by:

a. Nifedipine
b. Frusemide
c. Nitrates
d. Captopril
e. Prazosin

Q.5.3 Mitral valve prolapse is recognised to be associated with:

a. Marfan's syndrome
b. Acromegaly
c. Ventricular septal defect
d. Polyarteritis nodosum
e. Hypertrophic obstructive cardiomyopathy

Q.5.4 Cannon waves in the jugular venous pulse are a recognised feature of:

a. Atrial fibrillation
b. Pericardial effusion
c. Complete atrio-ventricular block
d. Ventricular pacing
e. Junctional (nodal) ectopic beats

Q.5.5 Which of the following are signs of portal hypertension:

a. Spider naevi
b. Caput medusa
c. Hepatomegaly
d. Splenomegaly
e. Ascites

Q.5.6 Anticipated complications of free gastro-oesophageal reflux due to hiatus hernia include:

a. Perforation into the mediastinum
b. Oesophageal carcinoma
c. Iron-deficiency anaemia
d. Recurrent aspiration pneumonia
e. Oesophageal stricture

Q.5.7 Recognised causes of constipation include:

a. Staphylococci
b. Hypothyroidism
c. Sarcoidosis
d. Enteric fever
e. Tricyclic antidepressant drugs

Q.5.8 Omeprazole:

a. Is an anticholinergic
b. Is a treatment for the Zollinger–Ellison Syndrome
c. Causes very high gastrin levels
d. Causes photo-onycholysis
e. Causes flatulence

Q.5.9 Recognised side-effects of danazol include:

a. Gynaecomastia
b. Optic neuritis
c. Hirsutism
d. Flushes
e. Haemolytic anaemia

Q.5.10 The angiotensin converting enzyme inhibitors (e.g. captopril and enalapril):

a. Are glycosaminoglycans
b. Are derivatives of proline
c. Have similar pharmacokinetics
d. May cause angioneurotic oedema
e. Inhibit the breakdown of bradykinin

Q.5.11 In hyperkalaemia:

a. Calcium-resonium may be indicated
b. Raised ST segments are often seen in the ECG
c. Cardiac arrest may occur in systole
d. There is an increased amplitude of the T-waves on the ECG
e. Intravenous etidronate is useful in treatment

Q.5.12 Recognised complications of alcoholism include:

a. Obstructive cardiomyopathy
b. Pancreatitis
c. Autonomic neuropathy
d. Hypoglycaemia
e. Coeliac disease

Q.5.13 Features of systemic lupus erythematosus include:

a. Proteinuria
b. Onychophagy
c. Photosensitive skin rash
d. Pleural effusion
e. Psychomotor retardation

Q.5.14 Recognised features of hypoglycaemia include:

a. Peripheral neuropathy
b. Paraesthesiae
c. Dyslexia
d. Hemiparesis
e. Aggressive behaviour

Q.5.15 Recognised sequelae of myocardial infarction include:

a. Infective endocarditis
b. Cerebral embolus
c. Septal perforation
d. Aortic aneurysm
e. Horner's syndrome

Q.5.16 Which of the following are normal haematological values in adults:

a. Basophils – < 0.1 × 10%/litre
b. Schilling test – > 10% of vitamin B_{12} dose excreted in urine in 24 hours
c. Haemoglobin F – 2%
d. Serum iron – 45–70 μmol/litre
e. Red cell mass (males) – 25–35ml/kg

Q.5.17 In relation to nebulised drug therapy:

a. Bronchodilators may exacerbate angina
b. Co-ordination of breathing is not required
c. Bronchodilators require dilution in water
d. Nebulisers can be prescribed on form FP10
e. Bronchodilators in asthma have replaced the use of prophylactic inhaled steroids

Q.5.18 Sleep apnoea is recognised to be complicated by:

a. Bronchospasm
b. Polycythaemia
c. Death
d. Enuresis
e. Low $P_a\ CO_2$ during attacks

Q.5.19 Characteristic features of pulmonary consolidation include:

a. Displacement of the trachea
b. Impaired percussion note
c. Expiratory wheezes
d. Inspiratory crackles
e. Reduced intensity of the breath sounds

Q.5.20 In bronchial asthma which of the following indicate a severe attack:

a. An elevated arterial $P_a\ CO_2$
b. Peak flow rate 120 litre/min
c. Production of copious bronchial secretions
d. Pulsus paradoxus of 20 mmHg
e. A quiet chest

Q.5.21 Recognised features of early, massive, acute pulmonary embolism include:

a. Raised jugular venous pressure
b. Left parasternal heave
c. Central chest pain
d. Hypotension
e. Excellent prognosis

Q.5.22 Recognised presentations of carcinoma of the bronchus include:

a. An epileptic fit
b. Increased pigmentation
c. Collapse of a vertebral body
d. Thyrotoxicosis
e. Horner's syndrome

Q.5.23 *Helicobacter pylorii* is:

a. A gram positive organism
b. Causative of an acute gastritis
c. A straight rod
d. The cause of duodenal ulcer
e. Eradicated by De-Nol and metronidazole in most patients

Q.5.24 Causes of diarrhoea include:

a. Carcinoid syndrome
b. Hyperparathyroidism
c. Thyrotoxicosis
d. Diabetes mellitus
e. Phaeochromocytoma

Q.5.25 An apical mid-diastolic murmur may be found:

a. In severe aortic regurgitation
b. In hypertensive heart disease
c. With a floppy mitral valve
d. In acute myocarditis
e. In mitral stenosis

Q.5.26 The jugular venous pressure:

a. Is best assessed in the internal jugular veins
b. Is raised in constrictive pericarditis
c. Is raised in tricuspid incompetence
d. Is raised in subarachnoid haemorrhage
e. Normally falls on expiration

Q.5.27 Atherosclerotic vascular disease is recognised to cause:

a. Aortic incompetence
b. Aneurysm of the descending aorta
c. Nocturnal diarrhoea
d. Elevated serum prolactin
e. A high systolic blood pressure

Q.5.28 Recognised features of severe acute left ventricular failure include:

a. Haemoptysis
b. Severe orthopnoea
c. Expiratory wheeze
d. Cough
e. Cold, clammy skin

Q.5.29 Lactic acidosis may be caused by:

a. Prolonged oxygen therapy
b. Uraemia
c. Alcohol abuse
d. Myeloproliferative disorders
e. Proximal renal tubular dysfunction

Q.5.30 Metabolic acidosis is a recognised feature of:

a. Methanol intoxication
b. Diuretic therapy
c. Ureterosigmoidostomy
d. Medullary sponge kidney
e. Aspirin overdosage

Q.5.31 Compared with a 30 year old woman, a 75 year old woman is more likely to develop:

a. Insulin dependent diabetes mellitus
b. Chronic lymphocytic leukaemia
c. Subdural haematoma
d. Temporal arteritis
e. Lupus pernio

Q.5.32 The binding of drugs to plasma protein may be increased:

a. After myocardial infarction
b. In Crohn's disease
c. In neonates
d. In the nephrotic syndrome
e. After burns

Q.5.33 Impotence is a recognised feature of:

a. Antihypertensive drugs
b. Tuberculosis
c. Leprosy
d. Depression
e. Hyperprolactinaemia

Q.5.34 Which of the following are recognised causes of a toxic confusional state:

a. Salicylate overdose
b. Cushing's syndrome
c. Normal pressure hydrocephalus
d. Hypocalcaemia
e. Myasthenia gravis

Q.5.35 Organic cerebral dysfunction manifests as:

a. Primary delusions
b. Facial tics
c. Geographical disorientation
d. Macropsia
e. Short term memory loss

Q.5.36 Which of the following are characteristic features of myasthenia gravis:

a. Episodic diplopia
b. Muscle fasiculation
c. Nasal regurgitation during eating
d. Severe morning weakness
e. Obstructive ventilatory defect

Q.5.37 Speech is characteristically affected by the following conditions:

a. Myasthenia gravis
b. Motor neurone disease
c. Left middle cerebral artery occlusion
d. Parkinson's disease
e. Bell's palsy

Q.5.38 In a complete 3rd nerve palsy:

a. There is a defect of facial sweating
b. The pupil will be small
c. There is loss of the temporal field of vision
d. The ptosis can be overcome by looking upwards
e. The eye will be deviated medially

Q.5.39 Unilateral visual loss is recognised to be associated with:

a. A frontal lobe tumour
b. Giant cell arteritis
c. Multiple sclerosis
d. Atheroma of the external carotid artery
e. Compression of the optic tract

Q.5.40 Is the pain of the following conditions paired correctly with their characteristic aggravating factors:

a. Pericarditis/aspirin ingestion
b. Duodenal ulcer/bending forward
c. Vertebral collapse/coughing
d. Cerebral tumour/straining at stool
e. Myocardial ischaemia/swallowing food

Q.5.41 Cerebral malaria:

a. Is treated with intrathecal quinine
b. Causes erythema multiforme
c. Should be treated only if the diagnosis is firmly established
d. Occurs only in the tropics
e. Has an insidious onset

Q.5.42 Hepatitis C:

a. Is caused by a single virus
b. Is never fulminant
c. Can progress to chronic liver disease
d. Can progress to a chronic asymptomatic carrier state
e. Can be prevented by vaccination

Q.5.43 An incubation period of less than one week is found in:

a. Hepatitis B
b. Hepatitis A
c. Meningococcal meningitis
d. Rabies
e. Syphilis

Q.5.44 Pyrexia of unknown origin (P.U.O.):

a. Is an illness of at least three weeks' duration
b. Is a temperature exceeding 38.3 °C on several occasions
c. Can usually be successfully treated in the community
d. May be due to Fabry's disease
e. May be due to pulmonary embolism

Q.5.45 Legionnaires disease:

a. May be contracted by drinking infected water
b. Has an incubation period of about three weeks
c. Is caused by a gram positive rod
d. Is best treated with tetracycline
e. Characteristically causes a leukopenia

Q.5.46 Which of the following are caused by gram positive cocci:

a. Toxic shock syndrome
b. Gonorrhoea
c. Erysipelas
d. Legionnaires disease
e. Diphtheria

Q.5.47 Which of the following are features of congenital syphilis:

a. Chancre
b. Nasal discharge
c. Gummata
d. Parkinson's teeth
e. Aortitis

Q.5.48 Recognised consequences of prolonged enforced immobilisation in bed include:

a. Hypotension
b. Urinary tract infection
c. Constipation
d. Hypercalcaemia
e. Peripheral nerve palsy

Q.5.49 Antihistamines:

a. Are effective in the topical relief of urticaria
b. Increase anti-muscarinic side effects of tricyclic antidepressants
c. Antagonise betahistine
d. Are safe in pregnancy
e. Those which are less sedating are poorly transferred across the blood/brain barrier

Q.5.50 Human insulins:

a. Have 10 amino acids different from bovine insulin
b. Have 1 amino acid different from porcine insulin
c. Have been responsible for decreasing diabetic retinopathy
d. Are less immunogenic than porcine insulins
e. Have been shown to alter the awareness of hypoglycaemia

Q.5.51 Drug induced photosensitivity:

a. May be due to immune mechanisms
b. The action spectrum of the photosensitiser rarely coincides with its absorption spectrum
c. May cause onycholysis
d. May cause pellagra
e. Occurs predominantly after light exposure in the UVD (400–700 mm) range

Q.5.52 In the treatment of depression in the elderly:

a. Tricyclics have been specifically and conclusively shown to be of benefit
b. Mianserin may cause blood dyscrasias
c. Maprotiline has fewer anticholinergic side effects than tricyclics
d. ECT is poorly tolerated
e. Monoamine oxidase inhibiters are never used

Q.5.53 The following are recognised associations:

a. Alactasia – titubation
b. Male infertility – *Micrococcus* infection
c. Bubonic plague – LCAT deficiency
d. Lactose intolerance – pinta
e. Bradykinesia – Still's disease

Q.5.54 Increased pigmentation of the skin is a characteristic feature of:

a. Simmond's disease
b. Acromegaly
c. Nelson's syndrome
d. Haemochromatosis
e. Wilson's disease

Q.5.55 Which of the following spinal levels and reflexes are correctly paired:

a. C5-6 – Biceps
b. S1 – Ankle
c. C7 – Triceps
d. L3-4 – Knee
e. L5 – Plantars

Q.5.56 Which of the following conditions have polygenic inheritance:

a. Hypertension
b. Achondroplasia
c. Menke's syndrome
d. Albinism
e. Pyloric stenosis

Q.5.57 The following are recognised causes of dementia:

a. Pellagra
b. HIV infection
c. Head injury
d. Cerebrovascular disease
e. Haemodialysis

Q.5.58 Caffeine is:

a. A cause of cancer of the pancreas
b. A cause of genito urinary cancer
c. Teratogenic in man
d. A cause of cancer of the breast
e. An important risk factor for ischaemic heart disease

Q.5.59 Hyposensitisation has been shown to be of no benefit in:

a. Atopic eczema
b. Allergic rhinitis
c. Wasp sting anaphylaxis
d. Urticaria
e. Allergic conjunctivitis

Q.5.60 The following dermatomes are correctly described:

a. T1 – anteromedial forearm
b. T2 – axillae
c. L1 – postero medial thigh
d. L2 – antero lateral thigh
e. L3 – knee

Answers

Examination 1

A.1.1
a. T
b. T
c. T
d. F
e. T

A.1.2
a. F
b. T
c. F
d. T
e. F

A.1.3
a. F
b. F
c. F
d. T
e. F

A.1.4
a. F
b. T
c. F
d. T
e. F

A.1.5
a. F
b. T
c. T
d. F
e. T

A.1.6
a. F
b. T
c. T
d. F
e. F

A.1.7
a. F
b. T
c. F
d. T
e. T

A.1.8
a. T
b. F
c. T
d. T
e. F

A.1.9
a. F
b. F
c. F
d. T
e. F

A.1.10
a. F
b. F
c. F
d. F
e. F

A.1.11
a. F
b. T
c. F
d. T
e. T

A.1.12
a. F
b. F
c. T
d. F
e. F

A.1.13 a. F
b. F
c. T
d. F
e. F

A.1.14 a. T
b. F
c. T
d. F
e. F

A.1.15 a. T
b. F
c. T
d. T
e. F

A.1.16 a. F
b. F
c. T
d. T
e. T

A.1.17 a. F
b. F
c. T
d. F
e. F

A.1.18 a. F
b. F
c. F
d. F
e. F

A.1.19 a. T
b. T
c. T
d. T
e. F

A.1.20 a. F
b. F
c. T
d. T
e. F

A.1.21 a. T
b. F
c. F
d. T
e. F

A.1.22 a. T
b. T
c. F
d. T
e. F

A.1.23 a. T
b. F
c. T
d. F
e. T

A.1.24 a. T
b. T
c. T
d. T
e. F

A.1.25 a. F
b. F
c. T
d. F
e. F

A.1.26 a. F
b. T
c. T
d. F
e. T

A.1.27 a. F
b. F
c. F
d. F
e. F

A.1.28 a. T
b. T
c. T
d. T
e. T

A.1.29 a. T
b. T
c. F
d. T
e. F

A.1.30 a. T
b. F
c. F
d. F
e. F

A.1.31 a. T
b. F
c. F
d. T
e. T

A.1.32 a. T
b. T
c. T
d. T
e. T

A.1.33 a. F
b. T
c. T
d. F
e. F

A.1.34 a. T
b. T
c. F
d. F
e. T

A.1.35 a. F
b. F
c. F
d. T
e. T

A.1.36 a. T
b. T
c. T
d. T
e. T

A.1.37 a. F
b. T
c. T
d. F
e. T

A.1.38 a. F
b. F
c. T
d. T
e. T

A.1.39 a. T
b. T
c. F
d. F
e. T

A.1.40 a. T
b. F
c. T
d. T
e. F

A.1.41	a.	T	**A.1.48**	a.	F
	b.	T		b.	T
	c.	T		c.	T
	d.	T		d.	T
	e.	F		e.	T
A.1.42	a.	F	**A.1.49**	a.	F
	b.	T		b.	F
	c.	T		c.	T
	d.	T		d.	F
	e.	F		e.	F
A.1.43	a.	F	**A.1.50**	a.	F
	b.	F		b.	F
	c.	F		c.	F
	d.	T		d.	F
	e.	T		e.	T
A.1.44	a.	T	**A.1.51**	a.	T
	b.	T		b.	T
	c.	T		c.	T
	d.	T		d.	T
	e.	F		e.	T
A.1.45	a.	F	**A.1.52**	a.	T
	b.	T		b.	T
	c.	T		c.	T
	d.	T		d.	T
	e.	F		e.	T
A.1.46	a.	F	**A.1.53**	a.	F
	b.	T		b.	F
	c.	F		c.	F
	d.	T		d.	T
	e.	T		e.	F
A.1.47	a.	T	**A.1.54**	a.	F
	b.	F		b.	F
	c.	T		c.	F
	d.	T		d.	T
	e.	F		e.	F

A.1.55	a.	T	**A.1.58**	a.	F
	b.	F		b.	F
	c.	T		c.	T
	d.	F		d.	T
	e.	T		e.	T
A.1.56	a.	T	**A.1.59**	a.	F
	b.	T		b.	F
	c.	T		c.	F
	d.	T		d.	F
	e.	T		e.	F
A.1.57	a.	F	**A.1.60**	a.	F
	b.	T		b.	F
	c.	F		c.	T
	d.	T		d.	F
	e.	T		e.	F

Examination 2

A.2.1
a. T
b. T
c. F
d. F
e. T

A.2.2
a. T
b. F
c. T
d. T
e. T

A.2.3
a. T
b. T
c. T
d. T
e. T

A.2.4
a. T
b. F
c. F
d. F
e. T

A.2.5
a. F
b. T
c. F
d. T
e. T

A.2.6
a. F
b. F
c. F
d. T
e. T

A.2.7
a. T
b. F
c. T
d. T
e. T

A.2.8
a. F
b. F
c. F
d. F
e. F

A.2.9
a. F
b. T
c. T
d. T
e. T

A.2.10
a. F
b. F
c. T
d. T
e. F

A.2.11
a. T
b. T
c. F
d. F
e. T

A.2.12
a. T
b. T
c. T
d. F
e. T

A.2.13 a. F
b. F
c. F
d. F
e. T

A.2.14 a. T
b. T
c. T
d. T
e. T

A.2.15 a. F
b. T
c. T
d. F
e. F

A.2.16 a. F
b. F
c. T
d. F
e. F

A.2.17 a. T
b. T
c. T
d. T
e. F

A.2.18 a. T
b. T
c. T
d. T
e. F

A.2.19 a. T
b. T
c. T
d. T
e. T

A.2.20 a. T
b. T
c. F
d. F
e. T

A.2.21 a. T
b. T
c. T
d. F
e. T

A.2.22 a. T
b. F
c. T
d. F
e. F

A.2.23 a. T
b. F
c. F
d. T
e. F

A.2.24 a. F
b. T
c. T
d. F
e. T

A.2.25 a. T
b. T
c. T
d. T
e. T

A.2.26 a. T
b. F
c. T
d. F
e. T

A.2.27	a. F b. F c. T d. T e. T		**A.2.34**	a. F b. F c. T d. F e. T	
A.2.28	a. T b. T c. T d. T e. F		**A.2.35**	a. T b. F c. T d. F e. T	
A.2.29	a. T b. T c. T d. F e. F		**A.2.36**	a. T b. T c. T d. T e. T	
A.2.30	a. T b. T c. T d. F e. F		**A.2.37**	a. F b. T c. T d. F e. F	
A.2.31	a. F b. T c. F d. F e. T		**A.2.38**	a. F b. F c. F d. F e. F	
A.2.32	a. T b. T c. T d. T e. T		**A.2.39**	a. F b. F c. T d. T e. F	
A.2.33	a. T b. F c. T d. T e. F		**A.2.40**	a. F b. F c. T d. F e. T	

A.2.41 a. F
b. F
c. T
d. T
e. T

A.2.42 a. T
b. T
c. T
d. T
e. T

A.2.43 a. T
b. T
c. T
d. F
e. T

A.2.44 a. T
b. T
c. T
d. F
e. F

A.2.45 a. T
b. T
c. F
d. F
e. F

A.2.46 a. T
b. F
c. T
d. T
e. T

A.2.47 a. F
b. T
c. F
d. F
e. F

A.2.48 a. T
b. F
c. T
d. T
e. F

A.2.49 a. T
b. T
c. T
d. F
e. F

A.2.50 a. F
b. F
c. T
d. F
e. F

A.2.51 a. T
b. T
c. F
d. T
e. F

A.2.52 a. T
b. T
c. F
d. T
e. F

A.2.53 a. F
b. F
c. F
d. F
e. T

A.2.54 a. F
b. T
c. T
d. T
e. F

A.2.55	a.	T	**A.2.58**	a.	T
	b.	T		b.	T
	c.	F		c.	T
	d.	T		d.	F
	e.	F		e.	T
A.2.56	a.	T	**A.2.59**	a.	F
	b.	F		b.	F
	c.	F		c.	T
	d.	F		d.	T
	e.	T		e.	F
A.2.57	a.	F	**A.2.60**	a.	T
	b.	T		b.	T
	c.	T		c.	F
	d.	F		d.	T
	e.	T		e.	F

Examination 3

A.3.1
a. T
b. T
c. T
d. F
e. F

A.3.2
a. F
b. F
c. F
d. T
e. F

A.3.3
a. F
b. F
c. F
d. T
e. T

A.3.4
a. T
b. T
c. F
d. F
e. F

A.3.5
a. F
b. T
c. T
d. T
e. F

A.3.6
a. F
b. T
c. T
d. F
e. T

A.3.7
a. T
b. T
c. F
d. F
e. T

A.3.8
a. T
b. T
c. T
d. T
e. T

A.3.9
a. T
b. F
c. T
d. T
e. F

A.3.10
a. T
b. F
c. F
d. T
e. F

A.3.11
a. F
b. F
c. T
d. T
e. T

A.3.12
a. F
b. F
c. F
d. T
e. F

A.3.13 a. F
b. F
c. F
d. F
e. F

A.3.14 a. F
b. F
c. T
d. T
e. T

A.3.15 a. F
b. F
c. F
d. F
e. T

A.3.16 a. F
b. F
c. F
d. F
e. F

A.3.17 a. F
b. T
c. F
d. T
e. T

A.3.18 a. F
b. T
c. T
d. F
e. T

A.3.19 a. F
b. F
c. F
d. T
e. T

A.3.20 a. F
b. F
c. T
d. F
e. T

A.3.21 a. T
b. F
c. F
d. F
e. T

A.3.22 a. T
b. F
c. T
d. T
e. F

A.3.23 a. T
b. T
c. T
d. F
e. T

A.3.24 a. F
b. F
c. F
d. T
e. T

A.3.25 a. T
b. F
c. F
d. F
e. F

A.3.26 a. T
b. F
c. F
d. F
e. T

A.3.27
a. T
b. F
c. F
d. T
e. T

A.3.28
a. T
b. T
c. T
d. F
e. F

A.3.29
a. T
b. F
c. T
d. F
e. T

A.3.30
a. F
b. T
c. T
d. F
e. T

A.3.31
a. T
b. F
c. T
d. T
e. F

A.3.32
a. F
b. F
c. T
d. F
e. F

A.3.33
a. F
b. T
c. F
d. T
e. T

A.3.34
a. T
b. T
c. F
d. T
e. F

A.3.35
a. F
b. T
c. F
d. T
e. T

A.3.36
a. T
b. T
c. F
d. T
e. F

A.3.37
a. T
b. F
c. T
d. T
e. F

A.3.38
a. F
b. F
c. T
d. F
e. T

A.3.39
a. T
b. T
c. T
d. F
e. F

A.3.40
a. T
b. T
c. T
d. T
e. T

A.3.41	a.	F
	b.	F
	c.	F
	d.	F
	e.	F
A.3.42	a.	F
	b.	T
	c.	F
	d.	T
	e.	T
A.3.43	a.	T
	b.	T
	c.	F
	d.	F
	e.	F
A.3.44	a.	F
	b.	F
	c.	T
	d.	T
	e.	F
A.3.45	a.	F
	b.	T
	c.	T
	d.	T
	e.	F
A.3.46	a.	F
	b.	F
	c.	F
	d.	T
	e.	T
A.3.47	a.	F
	b.	F
	c.	T
	d.	F
	e.	F
A.3.48	a.	F
	b.	T
	c.	F
	d.	T
	e.	F
A.3.49	a.	T
	b.	F
	c.	T
	d.	F
	e.	F
A.3.50	a.	F
	b.	F
	c.	T
	d.	F
	e.	F
A.3.51	a.	T
	b.	T
	c.	T
	d.	T
	e.	T
A.3.52	a.	T
	b.	T
	c.	T
	d.	F
	e.	T
A.3.53	a.	F
	b.	F
	c.	F
	d.	F
	e.	F
A.3.54	a.	T
	b.	T
	c.	T
	d.	T
	e.	T

A.3.55	a.	F	**A.3.58**	a.	T
	b.	T		b.	T
	c.	F		c.	F
	d.	F		d.	F
	e.	T		e.	T
A.3.56	a.	T	**A.3.59**	a.	F
	b.	T		b.	F
	c.	T		c.	F
	d.	T		d.	T
	e.	F		e.	F
A.3.57	a.	T	**A.3.60**	a.	T
	b.	F		b.	F
	c.	T		c.	T
	d.	T		d.	T
	e.	T		e.	F

Examination 4

A.4.1	a.	F	**A.4.7**	a.	F
	b.	F		b.	F
	c.	T		c.	T
	d.	T		d.	T
	e.	F		e.	T
A.4.2	a.	F	**A.4.8**	a.	T
	b.	T		b.	T
	c.	T		c.	T
	d.	T		d.	T
	e.	F		e.	T
A.4.3	a.	F	**A.4.9**	a.	F
	b.	F		b.	T
	c.	F		c.	T
	d.	F		d.	F
	e.	F		e.	F
A.4.4	a.	F	**A.4.10**	a.	F
	b.	F		b.	F
	c.	F		c.	F
	d.	F		d.	T
	e.	F		e.	F
A.4.5	a.	F	**A.4.11**	a.	T
	b.	T		b.	F
	c.	F		c.	T
	d.	F		d.	F
	e.	F		e.	T
A.4.6	a.	T	**A.4.12**	a.	F
	b.	F		b.	F
	c.	F		c.	T
	d.	T		d.	T
	e.	T		e.	T

A.4.13	a.	T	**A.4.20**	a.	F
	b.	T		b.	F
	c.	F		c.	T
	d.	T		d.	F
	e.	F		e.	T
A.4.14	a.	F	**A.4.21**	a.	F
	b.	F		b.	T
	c.	F		c.	T
	d.	T		d.	F
	e.	F		e.	T
A.4.15	a.	F	**A.4.22**	a.	F
	b.	F		b.	T
	c.	F		c.	F
	d.	T		d.	F
	e.	T		e.	T
A.4.16	a.	T	**A.4.23**	a.	F
	b.	T		b.	T
	c.	F		c.	T
	d.	F		d.	F
	e.	T		e.	F
A.4.17	a.	T	**A.4.24**	a.	T
	b.	F		b.	F
	c.	F		c.	F
	d.	T		d.	T
	e.	F		e.	F
A.4.18	a.	F	**A.4.25**	a.	T
	b.	T		b.	F
	c.	F		c.	F
	d.	T		d.	T
	e.	T		e.	T
A.4.19	a.	F	**A.4.26**	a.	T
	b.	F		b.	T
	c.	T		c.	T
	d.	T		d.	F
	e.	T		e.	F

A.4.27	a.	F	**A.4.34**	a.	T
	b.	T		b.	T
	c.	T		c.	F
	d.	T		d.	F
	e.	T		e.	F
A.4.28	a.	T	**A.4.35**	a.	T
	b.	T		b.	F
	c.	T		c.	T
	d.	F		d.	F
	e.	T		e.	F
A.4.29	a.	F	**A.4.36**	a.	F
	b.	T		b.	T
	c.	T		c.	T
	d.	T		d.	F
	e.	F		e.	F
A.4.30	a.	F	**A.4.37**	a.	T
	b.	F		b.	T
	c.	F		c.	T
	d.	F		d.	F
	e.	T		e.	T
A.4.31	a.	T	**A.4.38**	a.	T
	b.	F		b.	T
	c.	F		c.	T
	d.	T		d.	T
	e.	T		e.	T
A.4.32	a.	T	**A.4.39**	a.	T
	b.	F		b.	F
	c.	T		c.	T
	d.	F		d.	T
	e.	F		e.	F
A.4.33	a.	F	**A.4.40**	a.	F
	b.	F		b.	T
	c.	F		c.	F
	d.	T		d.	T
	e.	T		e.	T

A.4.41	a.	F	**A.4.48**	a.	F
	b.	T		b.	F
	c.	F		c.	T
	d.	F		d.	T
	e.	T		e.	F
A.4.42	a.	T	**A.4.49**	a.	T
	b.	T		b.	T
	c.	T		c.	T
	d.	T		d.	T
	e.	T		e.	T
A.4.43	a.	F	**A.4.50**	a.	F
	b.	F		b.	F
	c.	T		c.	F
	d.	F		d.	F
	e.	T		e.	T
A.4.44	a.	F	**A.4.51**	a.	T
	b.	F		b.	F
	c.	F		c.	F
	d.	T		d.	T
	e.	F		e.	F
A.4.45	a.	F	**A.4.52**	a.	T
	b.	T		b.	F
	c.	T		c.	F
	d.	T		d.	F
	e.	T		e.	T
A.4.46	a.	F	**A.4.53**	a.	T
	b.	F		b.	T
	c.	T		c.	T
	d.	F		d.	T
	e.	T		e.	T
A.4.47	a.	F	**A.4.54**	a.	T
	b.	T		b.	T
	c.	T		c.	F
	d.	F		d.	T
	e.	T		e.	F

A.4.55
a. F
b. T
c. F
d. T
e. T

A.4.56
a. F
b. T
c. T
d. T
e. T

A.4.57
a. T
b. T
c. T
d. T
e. T

A.4.58
a. F
b. T
c. T
d. F
e. F

A.4.59
a. T
b. T
c. T
d. T
e. F

A.4.60
a. F
b. T
c. T
d. T
e. F

Examination 5

A.5.1
a. T
b. T
c. T
d. T
e. T

A.5.2
a. F
b. T
c. T
d. F
e. T

A.5.3
a. T
b. F
c. F
d. T
e. T

A.5.4
a. F
b. F
c. T
d. T
e. T

A.5.5
a. F
b. T
c. F
d. T
e. T

A.5.6
a. F
b. F
c. T
d. F
e. T

A.5.7
a. F
b. T
c. F
d. T
e. T

A.5.8
a. F
b. T
c. T
d. F
e. T

A.5.9
a. F
b. F
c. T
d. T
e. F

A.5.10
a. F
b. T
c. F
d. T
e. T

A.5.11
a. T
b. F
c. F
d. T
e. F

A.5.12
a. F
b. T
c. F
d. T
e. F

A.5.13 a. T b. F c. T d. T e. T

A.5.14 a. F b. T c. F d. T e. T

A.5.15 a. F b. T c. T d. F e. F

A.5.16 a. T b. T c. F d. F e. T

A.5.17 a. T b. T c. F d. F e. F

A.5.18 a. F b. T c. T d. T e. F

A.5.19 a. F b. T c. F d. T e. F

A.5.20 a. T b. T c. F d. T e. T

A.5.21 a. T b. T c. T d. T e. F

A.5.22 a. T b. T c. T d. F e. T

A.5.23 a. T b. T c. F d. F e. T

A.5.24 a. T b. F c. T d. T e. F

A.5.25 a. T b. F c. F d. F e. T

A.5.26 a. T b. T c. T d. F e. F

A.5.27	a.	F	**A.5.34**	a.	T
	b.	T		b.	T
	c.	F		c.	F
	d.	F		d.	F
	e.	T		e.	F
A.5.28	a.	T	**A.5.35**	a.	F
	b.	T		b.	F
	c.	T		c.	T
	d.	F		d.	T
	e.	T		e.	T
A.5.29	a.	F	**A.5.36**	a.	T
	b.	T		b.	F
	c.	T		c.	T
	d.	T		d.	F
	e.	F		e.	F
A.5.30	a.	T	**A.5.37**	a.	T
	b.	F		b.	T
	c.	T		c.	T
	d.	F		d.	T
	e.	T		e.	T
A.5.31	a.	F	**A.5.38**	a.	F
	b.	T		b.	F
	c.	T		c.	F
	d.	T		d.	F
	e.	F		e.	F
A.5.32	a.	T	**A.5.39**	a.	F
	b.	T		b.	T
	c.	F		c.	T
	d.	F		d.	F
	e.	T		e.	F
A.5.33	a.	T	**A.5.40**	a.	F
	b.	F		b.	F
	c.	F		c.	F
	d.	T		d.	T
	e.	T		e.	F

A.5.41	a.	F	**A.5.48**	a.	T
	b.	F		b.	T
	c.	F		c.	T
	d.	F		d.	T
	e.	F		e.	T
A.5.42	a.	F	**A.5.49**	a.	F
	b.	F		b.	T
	c.	T		c.	T
	d.	T		d.	T
	e.	F		e.	T
A.5.43	a.	F	**A.5.50**	a.	F
	b.	F		b.	T
	c.	T		c.	F
	d.	F		d.	T
	e.	F		e.	T
A.5.44	a.	T	**A.5.51**	a.	T
	b.	T		b.	F
	c.	F		c.	T
	d.	T		d.	F
	e.	T		e.	F
A.5.45	a.	F	**A.5.52**	a.	F
	b.	F		b.	T
	c.	F		c.	T
	d.	F		d.	F
	e.	F		e.	F
A.5.46	a.	T	**A.5.53**	a.	F
	b.	F		b.	F
	c.	T		c.	F
	d.	F		d.	F
	e.	F		e.	F
A.5.47	a.	F	**A.5.54**	a.	F
	b.	T		b.	F
	c.	T		c.	T
	d.	F		d.	T
	e.	T		e.	T

A.5.55	a.	T	**A.5.58**	a.	F
	b.	T		b.	F
	c.	T		c.	F
	d.	T		d.	F
	e.	F		e.	F
A.5.56	a.	T	**A.5.59**	a.	T
	b.	F		b.	F
	c.	F		c.	F
	d.	F		d.	T
	e.	T		e.	T
A.5.57	a.	T	**A.5.60**	a.	T
	b.	T		b.	F
	c.	T		c.	F
	d.	T		d.	T
	e.	T		e.	T